Gays, AIDS and You

Gays, AIDS and You

Enrique T. Rueda
and
Michael Schwartz

THE DEVIN ADAIR COMPANY

OLD GREENWICH, CONNECTICUT

Copyright © 1987 by Devin Adair Company
Old Greenwich, Connecticut, 06870

Permission to quote from this volume must be obtained in
writing from the publisher, The Devin Adair
Company, Old Greenwich, Connecticut 06870.

Library of Congress Cataloging-in-Publication Data

Rueda, Enrique, 1939–
Gays, AIDS and you.

1. Gay liberation movement—United States.
2. Homosexuality—United States.   3. AIDS (Disease)—
United States.   I. Schwartz, Michael, 1949–
II. Title.
HQ76.8.U5R82   1987   306.7'662   87-24527
ISBN 0-8159-5627-4
ISBN 0-8159-5624-X (pbk.)

ABOUT THE AUTHORS

MICHAEL SCHWARTZ is Director of the Child and Family Policy Division of the Free Congress Research and Education Foundation in Washington, D.C.

The author of three books and hundreds of articles, Mr. Schwartz received the Thomas Linacre Award for excellence in medical-moral journalism in 1980. In that same year he was elected to the Wisconsin delegation to the White House Conference on Families.

REVEREND ENRIQUE RUEDA was founder and a Director of the Catholic Center at the Free Congress Research and Education Foundation, where he held a research fellowship. A native of Cuba, he was imprisoned by the communists during the Bay of Pigs invasion. Father Rueda has done extensive research and writing on Latin America in general and the current situation in Central America in particular. His several degrees include a Master of Arts in Political Science from Fordham University and advanced degrees in Divinity and Theology from St. Joseph's Seminary. He has served as a chaplain to migrant workers and college students, directed a drug abuse education center and done pastoral work in the South Bronx, New York. Father Rueda's previous publications include numerous monographs, a book-length work on drug abuse education and a scholarly book entitled *The Homosexual Network*. He writes a weekly column on public policy issues and is currently a Senior Contributing Scholar at the Catholic Center.

INTRODUCTION

This is not a medical textbook, with a detailed explanation of how the AIDS virus travels from one person to another and with instructions about how to avoid becoming infected. This is a report—in plain English—designed to show what the homosexual movement is, the power it wields and how it is using the AIDS epidemic to pursue its political agenda.

Why do *you* need to read this book? Because the homosexual political agenda represents a radical departure from what we as Americans believe. Once you understand the agenda of the homosexual movement, you will probably perceive it as a terrible threat—to ourselves, our children, our communities, our country. As a matter of fact, the homosexual movement has a radical, anti-family agenda that the majority of Americans reject overwhelmingly. In essence, the homosexual movement wants a country in which homosexual acts are accepted as a normal variant of human behavior, and in which homosexuality itself is accepted as an "alternative lifestyle." This movement wants you to believe that "Gay is good"; that homosexuality itself is not a matter of choice, not changeable, not an illness; that "coming out" is a desirable, even a laudable action; that homosexuality has no moral implications; and that opposition to homosexuality is wrong. Finally, the movement wants all Americans to accept homosexuals as just another "legitimate" minority—like Blacks, or Indians, or Jews, or people who are left-handed.

This movement is stronger, more widespread, more skillfully structured than most Americans realize. It reaches into our media, our political institutions, our schools, even into mainline churches. It has already come closer to achieving its goals that most American know. Today, throughout the United States, our children are being subjected to homosexual propaganda to an extent that would have been unthinkable just a few years ago. Moreover, this is being done in ways most of us consider to be repugnant. For the homosexual movement is nothing less than an attack on our traditional, pro-family values. And now this movement is using the AIDS crisis to pursue its political agenda. This in turn, threatens not only our values but our lives.

This is not a book about the way things *ought to be*, but about the way things *are*. We believe that homosexuality is a manifestation of the sinful condition that affects mankind and each man, and that homosexual behavior is gravely sinful by the very nature of reality. Nevertheless, we accept homosexuals completely as human beings and as children of God. Homosexuals are entitled to our love and concern. They are loved by God as much as anyone else. This we believe while affirming the disordered nature of their sexual condition and the evil nature of the acts this condition leads to, and while fully committed to the proposition that homosexuals should *not* be entitled to special treatment under the law. That would be tantamount to rewarding evil.

As you will see in the pages to come, we are writing here not about individual homosexuals, but about the homosexual movement. This is an important distinction, for it is the movement and its ideology that threaten us. And when we use the words "gay" or "prohomosexual" to describe an individual, a theory, an institution, or a piece of legislation, we mean that it promotes conditions that favor the practice of homosexuality, or a principle of the homosexual ideology itself. In short, the dangers that we face do not come from the individual who is homosexual, but rather from the movement that promotes homosexuality, from the ideology this movement has adopted, and from the movement's political and social goals for America. In essence, the danger we face today comes not from homosexuality, which is a *condition*, but rather from the *gay lifestyle* that some homosexuals pursue and advocate. Thus we do not condemn homosexuals as individuals, but rather the actions some of them are taking. Homosexual individuals struggling to overcome their disordered impulses deserve our support, praise, and friendship.

One warning before we begin: We have written this book as simply and as plainly as we can. You have a right to know what is happening in our country, what ideology is being imposed on your children, what threats we face. But to warn we must first describe, and some of what follows may be offensive or even repugnant. As you read through it, please keep in mind that today, all over America, our children are at risk. Our sole purpose in writing this book is to show you what you need to know to protect them, and by doing so protect yourselves, your communities, and our country.

CONTENTS

Gays, AIDS and You

CHAPTER ONE

'AIDS Is Our Strength!'

The AIDS plague in America is a result of promiscuous homosexual behavior.

Around 1980 physicians began to find cases of Kaposi's sarcoma among young male patients. This is a rare form of cancer previously found, as a rule, in elderly men. Researchers found that these younger patients had two things in common: their immune systems—the body's natural defense against infection—had been destroyed by some unknown cause; and they were homosexuals. This strange new disorder was named GRID, Gay Related Immuno-deficiency Disease.

Homosexual rights organizations resented this terminology, and when cases began to appear among non-homosexuals, the name of the disease was quickly changed to the more neutral-sounding AIDS, which stands for Acquired Immune Deficiency Syndrome. Besides homosexuals, three other groups were listed as "high risk" categories: intravenous drug users, hemophiliacs and Haitians. (Haitians were later dropped as a separate category when it was learned that those afflicted had engaged in homosexual behavior or were drug addicts. AIDS shows no preference for any race or nationality.)

The number of diagnosed AIDS cases has increased geometrically, from 200 in 1981 to 2000 in 1983 to 10,000 in 1985 to 40,000 in 1987. Worse still, researchers estimate that for every current case of diagnosed AIDS, there may be as many as 100 other persons who are infected with the lethal virus. No one has ever recovered from AIDS. Most die within two years of the appearance of diagnosable symptoms, although researchers estimate that it may take as long as five to fifteen years after infection for the symptoms to appear in an otherwise healthy infected person. During that entire time, the infected person can transmit the infection to others.

If AIDS had been introduced to America among any segment of society other than homosexuals, it probably would not have spread so widely so quickly. This is for three reasons. Active homosexuals are so astonishingly promiscuous that an infected individual might pass the disease on to as many as 500 sexual contacts within a year. The acts in which homosexuals engage constitute the most efficient means of transmitting the AIDS virus. And homosexual pressure groups have been powerful enough to block most serious efforts at containing the disease.

Rampant promiscuity among the initial pool of homosexual AIDS carriers caused the AIDS virus to spread like a chain reaction within the homosexual subculture. It is relatively common for drug addicts to resort to homosexual prostitution. AIDS was thus introduced into another subculture. The sharing of infected needles spread the disease throughout the drug addict population.

Both of these groups, active homosexuals and drug addicts, are defined by the deviant acts in which they engage. It could be said that their susceptibility to AIDS is a consequence of their behavior. But the next group to be stricken by AIDS was one which certainly could not be willfully exposing themselves to risk. They were hemophiliacs and other patients who were infected through transfusions of AIDS-contaminated blood and blood products that had been sold or donated by homosexuals and drug addicts.

When AIDS first began to appear among hemophiliacs, the National Hemophilia Foundation urged that homosexuals be prohibited from donating blood. This proposal was angrily denounced by the National Gay Task Force as "dangerous and divisive," and they accused the Hemophilia Foundation of seeking "a political solution to a medical problem." By 1987 three-fourths of the hemophiliacs in America were infected.

Because of the strong pressure brought by homosexual groups, the Centers for Disease Control neglected to advise homosexuals not to donate blood until 1983. As of this writing, it still does not prohibit blood donations from homosexuals.

The AIDS epidemic has continued to spread, especially among ethnic minorities. Bisexual AIDS carriers and infected drug users have spread the disease to women through sexual contact. Some of these women are prostitutes who by definition are also extremely promiscuous. Infected women have passed on the virus to children. Babies born to or nursed by infected women have become infected. Health care professionals have in some cases also been infected.

The number of documented cases of AIDS transmission by vectors other than sexual contact, sharing of needles, or blood transfusions is very small so far. But this does not mean that such transmission is impossible. Indeed, we know that it is possible because there are some of these cases on record. It is even possible that the number of such cases is larger than anyone now suspects because a person who is infected by some other means is not likely to be aware that infection has occurred, and may show no symptoms until years later.

The AIDS virus is present in the blood, saliva and tears of an infected person, even if that person shows no symptoms of the disease. This creates the frightening possibility that infection may occur accidentally. That is, of course, a very remote possibility, and public health officials might have allayed most of these concerns by acknowledging the risk levels in a realistic manner and proposing preventive measures that would reduce those risks even further. But the homosexual movement is unwilling to admit any risk at all of accidental transmission of AIDS and so, bowing to that pressure, most public health officials have simply repeated that accidental transmission is impossible. These denials stand in contradiction to the precautions taken by police officers, dentists and others whose occupations may expose them to the risk of accidental contact with infected body fluids. The result is an erosion in the credibility of public health officials and higher levels of public concern.

Even more frightening is the fact that the overwhelming majority of those who are infected do not know they are infected and may be passing the disease on to others. By the end of 1986, only 87,000 persons had tested positive for the AIDS virus, out of a total of 11.4 million tests. By far, the majority of these tests were of blood donors, among whom infection rates were extremely low. The next largest group was military personnel and recruits, among whom infection levels varied from one locality to another, but reached levels as high as 2 percent in some major urban areas. Voluntary testing programs had reached only small numbers of people.

At that same time, the Department of Health and Human Services estimated that 1.5 million Americans were infected with AIDS, and some private groups estimated that the number of cases may have been three times as high as the HHS estimate. If those estimates are reasonably accurate, then at least 94 percent, and possibly as many as 98 percent of the people who are infected with AIDS have not been tested and are unaware that they are carriers of the disease.

The question of testing became highly controversial in 1987 after President Reagan suggested, in a speech to an AIDS research foundation, that routine testing be instituted for certain categories of persons. The homosexual movement protested vigorously, even though homosexuals stand to gain the most from widespread routine testing because they are most at risk of infection.

This puzzling behavior in the name of the "rights" of homosexuals—opposition to testing and other public health measures, insistence on covering up important information about AIDS, demands that AIDS carriers be guaranteed the right to circulate freely in society—appears almost suicidal. Homosexuals, after all, have been the first group to suffer significant losses as the result of AIDS, and the AIDS plague is a threat to the life of every homosexual. A plausible explanation for this strange attitude is that gay rights leaders have not looked upon AIDS primarily as a health castastrophe, but as an opportunity to push forward their political agenda.

Although they deny it vehemently, the fact is that homosexual activists look upon AIDS as the "gay" disease. It seems to strike the homosexual subculture in a particular way, and even now 75 percent of the victims of AIDS are homosexuals.

AIDS has become for the homosexual movement an ideological source of strength: a shared suffering that creates a sense of solidarity, a special identity, and a justification for claiming the status of victim and for demanding the sympathy and, indeed, repentance of everyone else to atone for that victimization.

Understood in this sense, the slogan which has gained prominence in "Gay Pride" demonstrations and within the homosexual subculture, "AIDS Is Our Strength!," no longer seems so absurd. AIDS *is* a source of strength for marshalling homosexuals into active support for a particular, well-defined political agenda, while forcing the rest of society into acquiescing to that agenda.

This is why the homosexual movement has made AIDS the first politically protected disease in history.

Here's a brief outline of how this has happened. During the 1960s, and even more in the 1970s, a powerful network of homosexual groups was organized with the overall objective of gaining social legitimacy and legal approval for homosexual practices. Patterning themselves after the civil rights organizations that had successfully fought for legal protection against racial discrimination, this "gay rights" movement positioned homosexuals as a victimized minority persecuted by society at large for its "alternative lifestyle." Anyone who opposed the political goals of the "gay rights" movement, anyone who dared even to express moral opposition to homosexual practices, was accused of "homophobia," which gradually came to be viewed in some quarters as a wicked, perverse, ignorant prejudice; every bit as dishonorable as racism.

In about half our states, the movement secured the repeal of criminal statutes against sodomy. Even where these laws remained on the books, they were almost never enforced for fear of angry backlashes and accusations of "homophobia" against police, prosecutors, judges and legislators. Thus, even before AIDS had appeared the "gay rights" groups had won, either formally or informally, a legal "right" to engage in homosexual acts.

It was absolutely essential for these efforts to convince the public to accept three fundamental principles of the homosexual movement:

1) Homosexuals are born and not made. An individual's sexual orientation is innate, God-given, and absolutely beyond his or anyone else's control.

2) For someone who is, by nature, homosexual, it is entirely healthy and wholesome to act upon his sexual impulses and very unhealthy and psychologically dangerous to repress those impulses.

3) It is impossible for a homosexual to control his sexual impulses, and even more impossible for him to reverse his sexual orientation.

Every one of these assertions is scientifically untenable. Biologically and genetically, homosexuals seem to be the same as everyone else. There is no sound scientific evidence to support the claim that homosexuality is an innate trait; it is a psycho-sexual dysfunction not linked to any known genetic or biological factor. The universal trait of homosexuals is their desire to engage in sexual relations with members of their own gender.

It is possible for homosexuals to resist these desires. They, like everyone else, are endowed with free will, and with adequate social and personal support and a sincere desire to do so, they can achieve the difficult goal of gaining mastery over themselves and controlling their own sexual desires. As a matter of fact, a strong religious faith has proved helpful to many homosexuals in overcoming their impulses. In a number of other cases, it is possible for homosexuals to achieve complete freedom from their unnatural drives through appropriate psychotherapy. This is especially true among younger men who are not so deeply enmeshed in a behavioral pattern of yielding to impulses.

Nothing, therefore, is more dangerous to the individual homosexual than the ideology of the "gay rights" movement. The message of the "gay rights" movement is that it is hopeless to seek release from homosexual drives, and hopeless even to attempt to control one's own sexual desires. Since he has no choice but to enter ever more deeply into the pattern of homosexual behavior, he is encouraged on the one hand to idealize that homosexuality as normal behavior, and on the other to feel a deep resentment against society at large, which is portrayed as persecuting and insulting "gays" because it is too ignorant to appreciate the normality of homosexuality.

A crucial breakthrough for the homosexual movement was the decision of the American Psychiatric Association, at its 1973 convention, to remove homosexuality from the official list of psychiatric disorders. This gave an aura of legitimacy to the claims of the "gay rights" advocates, although, in fact, it was not a scientific statement at all. The declassification of homosexuality as a psychiatric disorder was very plainly the result of pressure tactics, intimidation and political manipulation.

This breakthrough was the turning point for the homosexual movement. Henceforth the ideology of the movement would be popularized by columnists, politicians and self-proclaimed experts. The ideological principle that homosexuality was normal fit in all too well with the temper of the times, as the sexual revolution of the 1970s led to a relaxation of publicly accepted standards of morality as well as the widespread popular feeling that whatever people did in private was no one's business but their own. Given that climate of opinion, the leadership of the homosexual movement began a concerted effort to extort a concession of legal and social legitimacy for homosexual behavior. In many localities, "gay rights" laws gave overt homosexuals special legal privileges in housing and employment. Homosexual pressure groups gained political prominence, and soon politicians were actively seeking their endorsement and support, and in return doing favors for the "gay rights" activists once they were in office. Most importantly, the practice of homosexuality became acceptable among the elites of our culture. In entertainment, in education, even in religion, homosexuality was often implicitly treated as a legitimate "alternative lifestyle" and self-confessed homosexuals became respectable company, not in spite of, but precisely because of, their homosexuality.

This aggressive attitude led many homosexuals to "come out of the closet," to acknowledge publicly their addiction to homosexual practices and to express their pride in being "gay." In virtually every major city, including those in which sodomy remained technically illegal, certain neighborhoods became "gay districts," with bars, bathhouses, bookstores, clubs, theaters and other commercial establishments catering to a homosexual clientele. Local homosexual newspapers and political organizations, as well as the appearance of gay-oriented art, literature and, of course, pornography, all helped to fashion a visible homosexual subculture.

Among the institutions that became necessary in that

subculture was a network of clinics treating sexually-transmitted diseases among homosexuals. The incredible levels of promiscuity and the unsanitary nature of the various ways in which homosexuals sought stimulation led to the epidemic spread of infectious diseases within the subculture.

In the early 1980s about half the cases of gonorrhea in the United States were occurring among homosexuals. Hepatitis B, which, like AIDS, is spread through the exchange of contaminated bodily fluids, is relatively rare in the United States except among homosexuals and drug addicts. In these two groups it is epidemic. Some studies suggest that over 90% of active homosexuals have had hepatitis B or other chronic or recurrent viral infections, including genital herpes and cytomegalovirus. Also prevalent among homosexuals are a variety of intestinal parasites, known collectively as the "gay bowel syndrome," and hepatitis A, which is spread through ingestion of fecal matter.

Thus, even before AIDS appeared, there was a critical problem of sexually-transmitted diseases within the homosexual subculture. Some researchers have theorized that the physical debilitation caused by repeated attacks of these infections has made homosexuals generally less resistant to AIDS, so that AIDS progresses more rapidly among homosexuals than among healthier people.

By the time AIDS became known, therefore, there already existed a complex set of organizations and institutions to provide services, support and political leadership on the AIDS issue for the homosexual subculture. The first organization specifically formed to address the AIDS issue was the Gay Men's Health Crisis, formed in New York in January, 1982. Its executive director, Mel Rosen, remains one of the leading "gay rights" spokesmen on the AIDS issue. In other cities, organizations were formed specifically to address the AIDS problem and the existing homosexual organizations made AIDS their top priority and their rallying point.

Even apart from its direct impact on the health of homosexuals, AIDS could easily have become the death knell of the homosexual movement. There were some perfectly obvious conclusions to be drawn about the appearance of a mysterious killer disease that was spread primarily through homosexual contact and was spilling out into the general population, and those conclusions would have reduced the homosexual movement to social and political oblivion.

Among the public health measures that might have been taken to prevent the spread of AIDS were the enforcement (and where necessary, the re-instatement) of anti-sodomy laws, the shutting down of bathhouses and "gay" bars, the elimination of special homosexual laws that have forced employers, landlords and educational institutions to extend special privileges to open homosexuals, and the open expression of social disapproval of homosexuality. Drug addicts, as a group, are less influential than homosexuals, and it is difficult to imagine that, if drug abuse instead of homosexual practice had been the primary means of transmitting AIDS, there would not have been a very strong crackdown on the drug traffic.

With the prospect of seeing all their influence wane, homosexual movement leaders had to find ways to reframe the issue and to turn it to their advantage. They started with an immediate advantage. While most Americans were still unaware of AIDs, or remained fairly unconcerned since they did not fit any of the "high-risk" categories, homosexuals were all frightened by the possibility that they might contract the disease. This fear served to unite and activate them as nothing had before.

With a united constituency behind them and no serious organized opposition, the homosexual leaders went to work turning a public health issue into a civil rights issue. Their mission was to convince the public that the gravest problem raised by the AIDS epidemic was not that of protecting the uninfected from contracting the disease, but that of preventing the scapegoating of homosexuals. Television programs and magazine feature stories repeated the theme that prejudice against homosexuals was holding back research efforts and feeding anti-gay demagoguery. The general impression created was the AIDS sufferers were the victims not of a virus, but of the dread evil of "homophobia."

Instead of focusing attention on preventing the spread of the disease, which might have meant restrictions on homosexual behavior, they went on the offensive by accusing the government of not investing enough money in research to discover the cause and develop a cure for AIDS. Paul Popham of the Gay Men's Health Crisis, for instance, complained that the government was deliberately dragging its feet in the area of AIDS research. "What I really think," he said, "is that it's the homophobia that's causing them not to go beyond the normal 'textbook" procedures, that they would go faster if they wanted to. If this happened to Boy Scouts, believe me, they would have found a way to get going."

Prohomosexual Congressman Henry Waxman (D-Cal.), echoed Popham's complaint. Early in 1982, when the public was first becoming aware of AIDS, he declared, "I want to be especially blunt about the political aspects of Kaposi's sarcoma. This horrible disease afflicts members of one of the nation's most stigmatized and discriminated-against minorities. The victims are not typical Main Street Americans. They are gays, mainly from New York, Los Angeles, and San Francisco. There is no doubt in my mind that if the same disease had appeared among Americans of Norwegian descent, or among tennis players, rather than among gay males, the response of both the Government and the medical community would have been different."

Public funding of AIDS research that year amounted to $5.6 million, although researchers hardly knew where to begin at that early stage of progress. In 1983 it was five times as high, and research funding went over the $100 million mark in 1985. No one has expressed opposition to medical research on AIDS, and research efforts have been amply funded and rapidly expanded. The issue Popham and Waxman raised was, in other words, a straw man, but their complaints helped draw attention away from the preventive efforts that might have been initiated at the same time.

It is true that the results of that research have been discouraging. It was not until 1983 that it was finally determined that a virus is the cause of AIDS, and not until 1985 that it became possible to test blood samples for the antibodies to that virus. Because of the nature of the disease, it seems theoretically impossible to produce a vaccine against it. A number of drugs have been developed that help alleviate the symptoms and prolong the lives of AIDS patients. But the prospect of finding a cure is remote. While research efforts obviously must be continued, it seems foolish to ignore effective preventive efforts while waiting for a major medical breakthrough.

AIDS education is another area in which federal, state and local levels of government have been generous, and here the homosexual movement has achieved significant successes.

The most obvious message of an AIDS education program would be to warn the public of the life-threatening nature of homosexual behavior. However, the homosexual movement successfully created the notion of "safe sex" as a way of preventing AIDS while preserving for its members the possibility of satisfying their sexual desires. It is not dangerous, they suggested, to engage in homosexual practices as long as a condom is used to protect against the exchange of body fluids. Public health officials, unwilling to risk charges of "homophobia" or moralizing, eagerly seized on "safe sex" as the way out of their dilemma. In fact, in relation to AIDS, "safe sex" is a contradiction in terms. Limited studies have indicated that condoms are not very effective in preventing the transmission of the AIDS virus. The only beneficiaries from the "safe sex" education campaign have been condom manufacturers who stand to make millions of dollars from the AIDS epidemic. Recommending "safe sex" is bad medical advice.

The only true form of safe sex is abstinence until marriage and fidelity within marriage. Although this is a fact, the homosexual movement has systematically thwarted the incorporation of this truth into AIDS education. The greatest triumph of the homosexual movement is the infiltration of homosexual ideas into the sex education courses taught in America's public schools. Hundreds of thousands of American students are now receiving detailed instruction in how to perform homosexual acts "safely." This, of course, is being presented in appropriately "non-judgmental" fashion, representing homosexual practice as one among many equally legitimate variants of sexual expression.

One obvious public health measure that would have had a positive impact on AIDS was shutting down the bathhouses and other commercial establishments that exist for the precise purpose of facilitating promiscuous homosexual activity. These places represent a clear public health hazard, and the Surgeon General has the legal authority to close them all. Still, neither he nor other public health officials in most localities have done anything to close these points for the distribution of AIDS. The way the homosexual leaders averted the closing of these establishments that have played a central role in the development of the homosexual subculture was to argue that the bathhouses provided an ideal setting for educating the at-risk population on the techniques of "safe sex." As the number of homosexual AIDS victims has increased, the forces of the market have caused many bathhouses to shut their doors. Many homosexuals found it so dangerous to patronize these establishment that they stopped visiting them.

Early on, when AIDS began to show up among hemophiliacs, it became evident that the blood supply needed to be protected.

In 1983, before blood screening was possible, "gay" activist Robert Schwab, now dead of AIDS, wrote in the *Dallas Gay News*, "if research money is not forthcoming at a certain level by a certain date, all gay males should give blood. . . . whatever action is required to get national attention is valid. If that includes blood terrorism, so be it."

Despite the known existence of this attitude among

some homosexuals, the Public Health Service did nothing more than issue an advisory later in 1983 "discouraging" homosexuals from donating blood. Dr. Selma Dritz, assistant health director for the City of San Francisco and a strong opponent of "homophobia," angrily denounced the suggestion that homosexuals should be forbidden to donate blood. "Flatly ruling out blood donations from an entire segment of society would be defamatory," she insisted.

To this day there are no laws or regulations prohibiting homosexuals from donating or selling their blood. To be sure, since 1985 blood donations have been routinely screened by the Red Cross and other private agencies for the presence of antibodies to the AIDS virus. This provides as high a measure of security as can reasonably be hoped for. *But thousands of Americans have already contracted AIDS from contaminated blood transfusions, in part because public health officials did not have the courage to offend the homosexual movement.*

In their public statements about AIDS transmission and preventive efforts, homosexual spokesmen have had to walk a fine line. On the one hand, they feel a need to minimize homosexual activity as a factor in spreading the disease, and so they have emphasized the possibility of transmission through heterosexual activity. This is, of course, a very real danger, especially among those who have sexual contact with bisexual men, drug addicts or prostitutes. Sexual promiscuity in general is very unhealthy, and not only because of the possibility of contracting AIDS. At the same time, it is necessary to recognize that the likelihood of even a highly promiscuous heterosexual person contracting AIDS is considerably less than that of becoming infected through homosexual activity.

The objective of the "gay rights" advocates in stressing the dangers of heterosexual transmission is to de-emphasize the role of homosexual activity in the spread of the disease, to popularize "safe sex" techniques as necessary for all persons to avoid infection, and above all, to imply a practical and moral equivalence between homosexual and heterosexual behavior. If "we are all in this together," then there is nothing peculiar about homosexuality.

At the same time, however, they find it essential to minimize, or even deny, the possibility of accidental transmission of AIDS. If it were recognized that AIDS can be acquired by other means than sexual contact, sharing needles or blood transfusions, then there might be a rational basis for uninfected persons to want to avoid contact with anyone likely to carry the AIDS virus. That would spell the end of the privileges for homosexuals embodied in "gay rights" laws, a fate which the homosexual movement feels must be avoided at all costs.

Serious arguments have been made for the thesis that AIDS can be transmitted accidentally. But calls for research to establish realistic risk levels and for the implementation of precautions to minimize those risks are denounced as irresponsible alarmism that will encourage "homophobia."

For example, in 1983 the *New England Journal of Medicine* published guidelines from the Task Force on AIDS at the University of California, San Francisco Medical Center, which included a caution about giving mouth-to-mouth resuscitation to AIDS patients. This led to complaints from a homosexual political group, and in response to that pressure the Task Force removed the caution from its guidelines. The argument of the homosexual organization was that this elementary precaution was "alarming" and that it encouraged "irrational or vague fears."

Health care personnel have, so far, been the group most vulnerable to accidental transmission of AIDS. However, there are instances in which nurses, orderlies and other non-physicians are not even permitted to know that a patient for whom they are caring is AIDS-infectious. In some institutions they have been forbidden to wear protective garments when treating AIDS patients, and AIDS patients are kept in the same wards as other patients, including children. From the perspective of the "gay rights" advocates, to treat AIDS patients in any way differently from others is discrimination rooted in "homophobia," even if the patient in question is not a homosexual.

Heterosexual AIDS victims make good test cases for the "gay rights" cause. Generally, the public is sympathetic to the plight of such persons, and if that individual can be secure in the "right" to attend school, retain employment, or otherwise continue to have contact with uninfected persons, then the chances of keeping "gay rights" laws and regulations on the books are that much stronger.

This effort received a major boost from the U.S. Supreme Court in March, 1987 when the Court ruled, in the *Arline* case, that persons with contagious diseases are included in the definition of the term "handicapped" as it is used in Section 504 of the 1973 Rehabilitation Act. Agencies and institutions that receive federal funds are prohibited from discriminating against "handicapped" persons. That anti-discrimination rule will now, presumably, apply to AIDS carriers. The plaintiff in that case was neither a homosexual nor an AIDS carrier, but a schoolteacher with chronically recurring tuberculosis. The Court ruled that her tuberculosis was not a *prima facie* reason for the local school board to remove her from a classroom teaching assignment. The ruling, was hailed as a victory by homosexual organizations.

It seems obvious that a program of widespread testing could help combat the spread of AIDS. Yet efforts to implement such a program have been systematically derailed by homosexual organizations.

The first reason in favor of routine AIDS testing is that everyone has a right and a responsibility to know if he is infected with the AIDS virus. That knowledge will enable the infected person to adjust his behavior so as not to endanger others, and to make the appropriate psychological, personal and social preparations for dealing with what may prove to be a terminal illness.

The second reason is that family members have a right to know that a member of their household is infected, so that they, too, can seek testing and take the necessary steps to avoid infection. Similarly, those with whom the infected person has had intimate contact will require testing.

A third reason is that physicians and other health care workers who are treating an AIDS carrier have a right to this information so that they can take the necessary precautions against becoming infected.

Finally, public health officials need this information so they can track the spread of the disease and direct their preventive and educational efforts to where they are most needed. Let's assume that in a high school a student is tested positive for AIDS. It would make sense to test all of the students in the class in order to find out how far the infection has spread, to inform the students that AIDS infection has been detected at their school, and to instruct them on what they must do to avoid infection. This is far more likely to have an impact on the behavior of these students than generalized exhortations to avoid sexual activity and drug abuse. Most importantly, it can save lives.

While widespread routine AIDS testing makes good sense to most Americans, homosexual groups have resisted it. They have gone so far as to publish editorials in homosexual newspapers urging readers not even to be tested voluntarily.

In the public arena, two main arguments have been advanced against routine testing. First, it is claimed that such testing is pointless since there is no cure for AIDS. While it is true that there is no cure, testing can be of great benefit in containing the spread of AIDS. Moreover, it is alleged that testing will result in persecution and discrimination against those who are infected. The only AIDS testing that homosexual groups accept is voluntary, anonymous testing so that no one except the person being tested will know if the test is positive. In California, where the homosexual movement is particularly powerful, this principle has been embodied in a law which prohibits a physician from informing anyone, even the spouse of an infected person, about the infection, despite the fact that withholding such information might cost the spouse's life.

It is, of course, possible, perhaps even likely, that if the names of AIDS carriers were published in the newspapers, they might be subject to unfair and inhumane treatment. But the ordinary standards of medical confidentiality preclude that possibility. Cases of gonorrhea must be reported to public health officials and must be followed up with contact tracing and testing. Most people who contract this disease would be embarrassed to have it publicly known, and some of them might face reprisals of some sort if that happened. But it does not happen. No one may have access to this kind of medical information except those who have a legitimate need to know. There is no reason to believe that the ordinary standards of medical confidentiality will not suffice to protect the privacy of AIDS carriers.

But there is evidence that treating AIDS testing information differently from other medical records is unsatisfactory. In Washington, D.C., AIDS test records were kept in a separate, high-security file, which was stolen in the spring of 1987. If they had been kept with all the other confidential medical records, such a theft would have been far less likely to occur. Instead of resorting to that sensible expedient, however, District of Columbia health officials decided not to keep records at all, and finally to discontinue testing.

The weakness of the stated reasons for opposing AIDS testing makes it reasonable to assume that there are unspoken reasons for explaining the intensity of homosexual activists concerning this issue.

One observer, a former homosexual who now operates a hospice for AIDS patients, speculates that, at bottom, the strong emotional opposition to testing is rooted in a fear of facing the possibility that one has AIDS. Many homosexuals, he says, realize that AIDS is something that can happen, but they are very unwilling to admit that it has happened to them. This is an understandable human reaction, and it might be a sufficient explanation of the problem.

Others have suggested that the opposition to testing is based on the expectation that widespread testing will reveal that AIDS infection is still overwhelmingly concentrated among homosexuals, and would thus upset the homosexual strategy of equating homosexual and heterosexual conduct as equivalent risk factors.

Whatever the reason, opposition to routine testing is clearly an impediment to any serious public health measures to contain the spread of the disease, and it is another indication of the degree of influence of homosexual activists over public health officials.

Closely related to the question of routine testing for public health purposes is that of testing by insurance providers. Many insurance companies, before writing a life or health insurance policy for an individual, will demand a physical examination and information about the individual's health habits. They sometimes charge higher premiums for persons who smoke cigarettes or who have high blood pressure. In some instances, they will refuse to provide coverage at all for those with a serious health problem. This helps to keep the cost of insurance lower for those who live in a healthier fashion.

Naturally, when the AIDS epidemic struck, some insurance companies demanded that potential clients be tested for AIDS infection. Homosexual groups charged that the insurance companies would use these test results to discriminate against those persons infected with AIDS. This should not be surprising since the whole point of the testing is to identify those who are at a higher risk on account of harboring the AIDS virus and treat them in a manner consonant with their condition. Insurance companies normally discriminate against smokers, cancer patients and other high-risk groups; or to put it the other way round, in favor of non-smokers and other healthy people. There is no reason why they should write insurance policies and charge the same rates for AIDS carriers as for those free of AIDS since the risks are not equal for those groups.

The charge of discrimination, with its implication of "homophobia," has led several jurisdictions, including the State of Wisconsin to prohibit insurers from requiring such tests. What happens then is plain to see from the experience of the District of Columbia, which passed an anti-testing ordinance in 1986. Forty-one of the top 50 insurance carriers stopped writing any new policies at all in the District of Columbia, and most of those which continued to do business there raised their premium rates. To protect AIDS carriers from "discrimination," residents of the District of Columbia now have to pay more for insurance and, even at those higher rates, have fewer insurance options to choose from.

For the leadership of the homosexual movement, stopping the spread of AIDS—at least within the non-homosexual population—is apparently not a high priority. As a matter of fact AIDS and the public concern over it is being used as a tool for winning public recognization of the legitimacy of homosexual conduct and for neutralizing those who object to such conduct. As the signs in the parades say, "AIDS Is Our Strength!"

How can such an attitude be explained? It is reasonable to assume that, except for what is related to their desire to engage in sexual relationships with members of their own sex, homosexuals are neither better nor worse than normal people. However, there is a streak of nihilism in the rhetoric of the homosexual movement. This nihilism has been strengthened by the existence of AIDS, a disease that has zeroed in on the homosexual population. Such nihilism affects individuals and the movement alike. For example, there are recorded instances of persons with AIDS who knowingly infected dozens, even hundreds, of others rather than alter their sexual practices. This would indicate, among some homosexuals, an almost violent resentment against normal society—a resentment which is encouraged within the homosexual subculture.

This resentment was given forceful expression in a guest editorial in the *Gay Community News* of February 15–21, 1987 by Michael Swift, "a gay poet and a gay revolutionary from Connecticut." He wrote:

> We shall sodomize your sons, emblems of your feeble masculinity, of your shallow dreams and vulgar lies. We shall seduce them in your schools, in your dormitories, in your gymnasiums, in your locker rooms, in your sports arenas, in your seminaries, in your youth groups, in your movie theater bathrooms . . . Wherever men are together . . . All laws banning homosexual activity will be revoked . . . If you dare to cry faggot, fairy, queer at us, we will stab you in your cowardly hearts and defile your dead, puny bodies . . . Be careful when you speak of homosexuals because we are always among you. . . . The family unit—spawning ground of lies, betrayals, mediocrity, hypocrisy and violence will be abolished . . . All churches who condemn us will be closed. Our only gods are handsome young men . . . All males who insist on remaining stupidly heterosexual will be tried in homosexual courts of justice and will become invisible men . . .
>
> We will demonstrate that homosexuality and intelligence and imagination are inextricably linked, and that homosexuality is a requirement for true nobility, true beauty in a man . . . Tremble, hetero swine, when we appear before you without our masks.

The author is surely not typical of all homosexuals. But the fact that such an effusion of hatred has been published by a "legitimate" newspaper within the homosexual community illustrates the reason why, at a time when civilization is threatened by AIDS, it is imperative that we take a look at the homosexual movement.

CHAPTER TWO

The Homosexual Movement

The homosexual movement exists at different levels. There are international, national, regional, and local organizations. Although its founders had from the beginning—as far back as 1924—a broad vision which encompassed *all* homosexuals, the strength of the movement lies in the fact that it is basically a grassroots movement.

The homosexual movement is the Wilde-Stein Club in Orono, Maine, and the Gay Nurses Alliance of Brownsville, Texas. The Alaska Gay Community Center, the Congregation Etz Chaim of Miami, and *The Community Voice* of the Wichita Gay Community Association are also the homosexual movement. The many congregations that make up the Universal Fellowship of Metropolitan Community Churches, the college-centered associations of homosexual students, the caucuses of professional homosexuals, the thousands of publications—from one-page newsletters to *The Advocate* and *The Sentinel*—are also the homosexual movement.

At the national level there are organizations that promote the homosexual ideology forcefully and effectively. For each national organization, however, there are dozens of smaller groups that work (most of them quietly, some with noise and fanfare) to ensure that the pressure of the "liberated" homosexual is felt throughout the land.

Within the movement, there are businesses (bars,

baths, bookstores, movie houses, and so forth), services (doctors, dentists, realtors, movers, counsellors, and others) and nonprofit organizations.

Although the homosexual movement can be described as a set of institutions, such a description provides an incomplete view. This is because the relations among groups, and the various ways in which individuals participate in the life of these institutions, is as important as the institutions themselves. In a sense, the homosexual movement is a nationwide network of interested individuals who have associated with each other for the promotion of an ideology that satisfies their own interests, both theoretical and practical. So when looking at the movement, it is essential to consider its networked nature in two ways. First, the leadership of the movement is made up of individuals who form a real network, usually acting in concert and often participating in various organizations within the entire network. Second, homosexual organizations do in fact act together, share information, and support one another. This is based on their shared interest—promotion of the homosexual ideology—and in the communality of their leadership. Moreover, in many instances the homosexual movement has successfully "infiltrated" other organizations. This provides additional platforms for the pursuit of common interests.

Although there is considerable networking activity at the national level, the homosexual movement works best at the local level. The movement is basically a grassroots operation. Especially in areas where there are large concentrations of homosexuals, in bars, baths, and even church groups, the practice of homosexuality and its perceived "value" for the psychosocial development of its devotees becomes entrenched in the minds of the "liberated" homosexual. Moreover, the importance of local groups and the need to recruit at the local level have not escaped the movement's national leadership. Many associations of homosexual college students have been formed with the help of the Gay Academic Union. The National Gay Task Force has a National Community Organizing Program, with a full-time staff person responsible for developing new homosexual organizations.

Efforts to organize homosexuals on the local level have resulted in some 3,000 organizations. San Francisco alone, for example, has a homosexual telephone directory listing some 600 businesses owned or managed by homosexuals, largely catering to a homosexual clientele. These include roughly a dozen legal services, a dozen medical services, a dozen religious organizations, along with some political organizations and real estate businesses. In New York the Greater Gotham Business Council has 100 members, presumably all homosexual businesses.

The homosexual movement is not limited to the United States. In a world where communications bridge thousands of miles in seconds and millions of people travel across international borders, no social development of the magnitude of the homosexual movement can be isolated. Homosexuals exist in all societies. The homosexual ideology, on the other hand, seems to be limited to Western nations. The Socialist bloc holds fast to the belief that homosexuality is a perversion, destructive of society. Its totalitarian governments have not allowed the development of anything remotely similar to the American homosexual movement. Although Moslem societies have traditionally been alleged to tolerate widespread homosexuality, the prevailing Moslem faith would not allow the existence of homosexual organizations.

There are well-defined homosexual organizations in Western nations. Representing twenty-one countries, national homosexual organizations have formed the International Gay Association (IGA). The IGA was organized in Coventry, England in 1978 by representatives of twelve countries. More recently up to twenty-one nations were represented with "associate" members in fifteen other countries including Austria, Brazil, Colombia, India, Indonesia, Japan, and Mexico. The main activities of the IGA are directed toward cooperation with the World Council of Churches (support for homosexual rights); Amnesty International (status for homosexuals in jail as "prisoners of conscience"); the World Health Organization ("deletion of homosexuality from its list of diseases and mental defects"); and other international bodies such as the United Nations and the Council of Europe.

Some of the activities and concerns of the IGA can be seen from the agenda of its First Annual Conference, held in the Netherlands in 1979. The topics discussed included "the status of lesbians and gay men around the world with respect to immigration and citizenship, child custody, persecution for engaging in homosexual acts, prison conditions, children's rights, education, and possible sources of support such as Amnesty International, the U.N., and the World Council of Churches."

Here in the United States, there are only three truly national organizations of the homosexual movement: the Gay Rights National Lobby (GRNL), the Universal Fellowship of Metropolitan Community Churches (UFMCC), and the National Gay and Lesbian Task Force

(NGLTF), which was originally known as the National Gay Task Force. There are other organizations that do not specifically relate to local issues and that, on this account, can also be called "national." However, they have neither the resources nor the influence to truly deserve this title. Of the other two, the NGLTF is older, more respected, and far more influential.

The NGLTF was founded in 1973 as a successful effort to heal a rift between moderate and radical homosexual leaders in New York City. Its board of directors includes some of the most influential persons in the movement itself.

The NGLTF's accomplishments on behalf of homosexuality have already left a deep and not easily erasable mark on our national life and culture. It was due to the efforts of the NGLTF that the American Psychiatric Association officially took homosexuality off its list of mental illnesses. The NGLTF was also instrumental in making the White House accessible and willing to lend a favorable ear to the leadership of the homosexual movement during the Carter Administration. This and the introduction of several prohomosexual statutes in the U.S. Congress—to a great extent also the work of the NGLTF—show the high degree of acceptance of homosexuality by the U.S. government itself. The high visibility of homosexual issues and personalities at the White House Conference on Families and the International Women's Year Conference was also due to the efforts of the NGLTF, as was the presence of prohomosexual individuals and agenda items at the 1980 Democratic Convention.

In addition, the NGLTF has been influential in causing a number of U.S. agencies—including the Internal Revenue Service, the Bureau of Prisons, and the Federal

Communications Commission—to make regulatory decisions which favor the acceptance of homosexuality as a legitimate lifestyle. Yet another area in which the NGLTF has been active is the promotion of the homosexual ideology in corporations by the adoption of "homosexual rights" policies. Finally, the NGLTF has secured support for the homosexual movement from dozens of organizations which could have been expected to remain "neutral" at best, among them the Young Women's Christian Association, the National Organization for Women, the American Civil Liberties Union, the National Council of Churches, and the National Federation of Priests Councils.

The NGLTF is basically a political organization. Its activities encompass three areas: 1) exertion of legal, legislative, and political pressure on the government, corporations, unions, and other organizations to "persuade" them to institute prohomosexual policies; 2) propaganda activities on behalf of the homosexual movement and in support of its ideology, especially in, but not limited to, the media; 3) grassroots organization, on both geographical and interest bases. The NGLTF acts to initiate small groups of homosexuals within "straight" organizations, with the specific aim of using the resources of these organizations on behalf of the goals of the homosexual movement.

The importance of schools in the promotion of any idea is obvious. Education is not only the most powerful "business" from an economic point of view, but the educational establishment views itself as the repository of the national ethos and the privileged elite responsible for molding our children. Not surprisingly, the homosexual movement has devoted considerable efforts to establishing an effective presence within academia. These efforts have paid off handsomely in terms of numbers, recognition, and influence.

For example the Gay Academic Union (GAU), incorporated in New York for the "advancement of gay studies," is organized on the basis of local chapters. There are fully charted units in Los Angeles, San Diego, San Francisco, Dallas, St. Louis, Chicago, Cincinnati, Greensboro (North Carolina), and Boston. These and other chapters appear to be well organized and active. For example, the San Diego chapter has ten semi-autonomous special interest groups (SIGs), among them the Arts and Entertainment SIG, the Artists' SIG, Research and Education SIG, and so forth. It also maintains a scholarship fund.

A central activity of the GAU is the promotion of the homosexual ideology on college campuses via university-based groups of homosexual students and faculty members. The very title of a publication of the GAU designed to accomplish this objective is quite revealing: "How to Infiltrate Your Groups." This manual was reportedly prepared with the advice of the American Civil Liberties Union.

Throughout the U.S., homosexual student organizations work on college campuses to channel student activism for the support of homosexuality. It has been pointed out that between one-half and one-third of local jurisdictions having prohomosexual legislation are college towns. Funding is apparently no problem for homosexual student organizations. Many schools actually finance the activities of prohomosexual groups from their student activity funds.

In fact there are many homosexual groups in American colleges and universities; they account for some twenty percent of all the homosexual organizations in the United States. A listing of college or university-related homosexual organizations would go on for pages, and it is apparent from even a cursory study that today in the U.S. almost every major college campus features at least one prohomosexual group. *The homosexual movement has thus succeeded in ensuring that the future American intellectual elite has been exposed to the homosexual ideology during its key, formative years.*

At the elementary and secondary level, the homosexual ideology is not promoted by the students themselves. However, homosexual teachers are well organized in certain areas of the country. including the following:

Boston Area Gay and Lesbian School Workers	Boston, Mass.
Gay Educators Association	Denver, Colo.
Gay Teachers Coalition	San Francisco, Calif.
Gay Teachers of Los Angeles	Los Angeles, Calif.
Gay Teachers of Maryland	Baltimore, Md.
Gay Schoolworkers	Ann Arbor, Mich.
Gay Teachers Association	New York, N.Y.

According to the Gay Teachers Association of New York City, there are up to 10,000 homosexual teachers in New York City alone. The following list of goals set forth by this organization reveals the way in which organized homosexual teachers promote their sexual proclivities. Should these goals be accomplished, it would be much easier for homosexual actions and homosexuality itself to be accepted by students, administrations, and faculties alike:

1. To provide a setting in which gay teachers can meet, share problems and ideas, and give each other support.

2. To conduct continuous negotiations with the New York City Board of United Federation of Teachers to obtain contractual guarantees of the right of gay teachers to teach in the city's public schools.

3. To work for the retraining of school administrators, teachers, and guidance personnel to enable them to meet the needs of gay students for counseling and support.

4. To promote curriculum change in all subject areas to enable gay and non-gay students to gain a realistic and positive concept of current gay lifestyles and the historic contributions of gay people.

5. To lobby as a teacher organization for the gay rights bill.

Bear in mind that the "current gay lifestyles" mentioned in Item 4 would logically involve transgenerational sex (i.e., child/adult sex), sadomasochism, homosexual prostitution, promiscuous sexual liaisons as seen in bars and baths, pornographic movie houses, and more. These practices not only seem to be intrinsic to the "current gay lifestyles" but are verified by the most casual examination of the average homosexual newspaper. Item 4 basically proposes a revision of curricula across the board—that is, in all subjects and grades—to make the schools promote homosexuality and clearly implies censorship of class material to fit the ideology of the homosexual movement. It is at least questionable whether most parents would appreciate a curriculum that would help their children develop a "realistic and positive concept" of sadomasochism, homosexual prostitution, or man/boy love.

A homosexual organization for librarians—who obviously have a great deal of influence on the intellectual formation of our children, is the Gay Task Force of the American Library Association, Social Responsibilities

Round Table division. This organization, launched back in 1970, was the first openly gay subgroup in a professional association. The Task Force is active in promoting the homosexual ideology through libraries. By its own admission, its members "work to get more and better gay materials into libraries and out to users, and to deal with discrimination against gay people as librarians and library users.

The Gay Task Force's preoccupation with the indoctrination of young people in the tenets of the homosexual ideology became apparent in the program for its 1975 conference. This program was entitled "The Children's Hour: Must Gay Be Grim for Jane and Jim?" The Task Force distributes bibliographies used by homosexual activists to ensure that publications favorable toward homosexuality are available in public libraries, including school libraries. See Figure 1 for a reproduction of the "core collection list" recommended by the Task Force in 1980.

As you can see, none of these books presents homosexuality in a critical or objective fashion. And some of the listed publications, such as the *Gayellow Pages*, contain drawings which are highly sexually suggestive and would probably be found offensive by most library patrons.

In addition to its academic-oriented groups, the homosexual movement has formed associations and organizations in just about every facet of American society. The variety of these associations and organizations—even at the national level—is so great that it is simply not possible to describe or catalogue them all. We will just describe some of them to provide a proper perspective on the true nature of the homosexual movement in our country today. Some of the most important prohomosexual

Gay Materials Core Collection List

Standard collection development tools such as H.W. Wilson's PUBLIC LIBRARY CATALOG have failed to reflect publishing trends with respect to gay materials. So we offer this list as a recommended core collection of non-fiction gay materials for small and medium size public libraries. We think college libraries also will find this basic list useful.

Books

Berzon, Betty and Robert Leighton, editors. Positively Gay. Celestial Arts, 1979.

Brown, Howard. Familiar Faces, Hidden Lives: The Story of Homosexual Men in America Today. Harcourt Brace Jovanovich, 1976; Harvest.

Curry, Hayden and Denis Clifford. A Legal Guide for Lesbian and Gay Couples. Addison-Wesley, 1980.

Fairchild, Berry and Nancy Hayward. Now That You Know: What Every Parent Should Know About Homosexuality. Harcourt Brace Jovanovich, 1979.

Hanckel, Frances and John Cunningham. A Way of Love, A Way of Life: A Young Person's Introduction to What It Means to Be Gay. Lothrop, Lee & Shepard (Morrow), 1979.

Jay, Karla and Allen Young, editors. After You're Out: Personal Experiences of Gay Men and Lesbian Women. Links, 1975; Pyramid.

McNeill, John J. The Church and the Homosexual. Sheed Andrews & McMeel, 1976; Pocketbooks.

Richmond, Len with Gary Noguera, editors. The New Gay Liberation Book. Ramparts, 1979.

Scanzoni, Letha and Virginia Ramey Mollenkott. Is the Homosexual my Neighbor? Another Christian View. Harper and Row, 1978.

Vida, Ginny, editor. Our Right to Love: A Lesbian Resource Book. Prentice-Hall, 1978.

Weinberg, George. Society and the Healthy Homosexual. St. Martins, 1972; Anchor.

Pamphlets and Directories

About Coming Out. National Gay Task Force, 80 Fifth Ave., New York, N.Y. 10011, 25¢ plus SASE; also bulk rates.

A Gay Bibliography. Gary Task Force, American Library Association, 6th edition March 1980. Selective non-fiction list of 563 books, articles, pamphlets, periodicals, directories, films. $1 prepaid from "Barbara Gittings—GTF" at address below; also quantity rates.

Gay Civil Rights Support Packet. Statements from groups in science, government, religion, health, etc. Natl' Gay Task Force, 80 Fifth Ave., New York, N.Y. 10011, $2.50 prepaid.

Gay Rights Protections in U.S. and Canada. List of law changes, revised quarterly. Natl' Gay Task Force, 80 Fifth Ave., New York, N.Y. 10011, 25¢ plus SASE; also bulk rates.

Gayellow Pages. Classified directory of gay/lesbian organizations, businesses and services in U.S. and Canada. Renaissance House, Box 292 Village Station, New York, N.Y. 10014, $8.50 prepaid.

Religious Support Packet. List of churches, officials and groups in religion that support gay rights. Natl. Gay Task force, 80 Fifth Ave., New York, N.Y. 10011, $3.00 prepaid.

Gay Task Force, American Library Association (Social Responsibilities Round Table) Box 2383, Philadelphia, PA 19103. Coordinator: Barbara Gittings (215) 471-3322.

FIGURE 1
Collection of Pro-Homosexual Materials Recommended by a Unit of the
American Library Association.

organizations are the more than 100 groups of parents and friends of homosexuals across the U.S. These groups have their common origin in the Parents of Lesbians and Gay Men, Inc., founded in New York City in the early 1970s. In 1979 the National Federation of Parents and Gays was founded in Washington, D.C.

The importance of these organizations, and other like them which have sprung up across the country, cannot be underestimated. Their existence and their activities strike at the very root of family life as it has been traditionally conceived in the U.S. Together with religion, the family has been at the forefront in defending the value of male/ female relations as part of the natural order and pro-claiming the intrinsic disorder of all other relations as inimical to the good order of family and society. Parents of homosexuals traditionally deplored the condition that affected their children, expressing shame and disgust at their "perverse" choice. By their nature, these organizations advocate the homosexual ideology by having some of these very parents support, applaud, and express pride in their children's heretofore condemned tendencies.

The homosexual movement does not consist of a ragged band of poor and oppressed individuals who are simply reacting with great rage and in anarchical fashion to unbearable injustice. Such a vision is carefully designed and nurtured to elicit the support of other Americans who have historically been part of groups that fit such a description. In truth, however, the homosexual movement represents large numbers of well-educated middle- and upper-class people. It has a coherent ideology and a vision of the future for America. The movement has created a subculture which represents the seeds of future growth. This subculture encompasses some institutions which are solely designed to satisfy the needs of the homosexuals. Other homosexual organizations exist within other larger institutions. They are merely means by which the movement attempts to convert host institutions into tools for satisfying its sociopolitical needs, or perhaps to "homosexualize" such institutions completely, making them integral parts of the movement.

The homosexual caucus within a church, for example, might work to make the homosexual ideology part of the tenets of the host church. This might be so repugnant to the traditional faith of the church that it is at best a long-range project. In the short run, it might suffice the goals of the movement to have the church implement elements of the prohomosexual movement such as:

—affirmative action with regard to homosexuals in its employment practices;

—incorporation of inclusive language in the services and/or sacred writings;

—the ordination of females—especially female homosexuals—by those churches whose doctrines have traditionally prescribed male clergy only;

—recognition of the church's homosexual groups as "legitimate" religious organizations;

—support for prohomosexual legislation.

The homosexual ideology implies the intent to rearrange our perceptions, lifestyles, and legal system. In the strict sense of the term, this change is revolutionary. It requires, if it is to be effecively implemented, the careful and gradual application and transfer of power. The homosexual movement is thus not primarily a philanthropic or educational enterprise, but a hard-nosed political movement bent on changing our society.

The homosexual movement understands well that the key to its success lies in its ability to influence—and ultimately control—policymakers. In several cases, the movement has been extremely successful in its ability to influence political structures. Washington, D.C. is a prime example of a jurisdiction in which the homosexual movement has maximized its political clout. For example, in 1978 Mayor Marion Barry—he is still the mayor in 1987—was elected with overwhelming support from the homosexual community. The 21 precincts where the homosexuals are concentrated—which represent 15 percent of the total electorate—gave 56 percent of their votes to Barry in the Democratic primary (the rest of the city voted only 30 percent for Barry.) It is estimated that of 5,000 homosexual votes, Barry carried 4,000. Homosexual bars staged pro-Barry fundraisers, joining the strictly political leadership in an all-homosexual effort to elect this liberal Democrat. Marion Barry has not forgotten that he is beholden to the homosexual leadership, and it is generally acknowledged that the homosexual movement has considerable input in major city-hall decisions, especially those affecting its interests.

Influencing policymakers throughout America is accomplished primarily through the ballot box. On April 21, 1980, a Congressional briefing was held in support of prohomosexual legislation, at which homosexual movement national leader Virginia Apuzzo pointed out the value of the homosexual vote:

> I am confident in telling you today that, despite your possible concern for your political future if you support civil rights for Gays, you have much more to gain by helping us than you have to lose. For every voter who may vote against you because of it there will be many times more who vote

for you because of it. We are 20 million strong and growing stronger. We have friends and family who love us and will stand with us. An attack on us will be seen as an attack on them, as well. We are good allies to have.

The political action of the homosexual movement also takes the form of pressure on existing parties to obtain their support for homosexual objectives. The movement achieved considerable success during the 1980 Democratic Convention by electing a significant number of homosexual delegates and having issues of importance to the movement made part of the party's platform. Similar, although much less successful efforts were undertaken within the Republican Party. Steve Stahl, Christian Social Action Co-chairman of the Metropolitan Community Church of Detroit, testified on homosexual affairs before the Republican National Platform Committee. Being allowed to testify was in itself a form of recognition and acceptance of the homosexual movement as a legitimate political force. Stahl made the following report:

> I was well received by the committee and I felt that a strong blow was struck for Lesbian/Gay rights. After a brief oral statement recounting the Democrats' involvement in rights issues, I challenged the Republican Party to prove their interest in the rights of the nation's minorities.
>
> Undoubtedly (*sic*) they will be slow to action, but I feel that they are awakening to the realities of the '80s. We must continue to apply pressure on the Republican Party and be prepared to "work" them against the Democrats. Both parties are keenly aware of the potential voting bloc our community represents.

Bear in mind again that the homosexual movement is not representative of poor people. In point of fact, it represents a group whose income is clearly above the national average. Moreover, even in a purely organizational sense—rather than as individuals—the various components of the homosexual movement have large sums of money at their disposal. This is translated into both individual contributions by homosexual activists to candidates who favor (or are expected to favor) homosexual legislation, and contributions collected by homosexual organizations. In November 1979 the National Convention Project sponsored a "Gay Vote USA Gala," a fundraising event in which the three leading Democratic candidates for the 1980 election—Jerry Brown, Ted Kennedy, and Jimmy Carter—were represented. The considerable funds collected were used to further the political interest of the homosexual movement, while serving the candidates who were responsive to the call of the homosexuals with the opportunity to court their votes while expressing varying degrees of support for their ideology.

In that same year the homosexual-oriented Municipal Election Committee in Los Angeles had reportedly raised $200,000 for local candidates alone, while the National Convention Project had at its disposal some $100,000 to influence the major parties. The impact of these homosexual dollars on the political process must not be underestimated, since they have money and, as a rule, political candidates are known to lend a friendly ear to their contributors.

The homosexual movement exerts its political clout in many other ways. For example, the Harvard Law School has bowed to the pressure of the homosexual movement—exercised through the Harvard-Radcliffe Gay Students Association—so that only law firms which agree not to consider homosexuality as a factor in employment are allowed to use the university's placement service for employment interviews. In this way, the movement accomplishes three objectives. First, an organizational component of the movement manifests its political clout. Feeding upon itself, this power gives its members and those affected by it the perception that the movement is not only real but productive. In other words, "nothing succeeds like success." Second, it makes a large and prestigious university a servant of the goals of the homosexual movement and an agent in the imposition of the homosexual ideology on the rest of society. Third, it transforms law firms into agents of the homosexual movement by making homosexuality acceptable as a lifestyle. This is a masterful use of the political power of what is probably a small group of students, and perhaps faculty members, in enrolling the support of powerful and respected institutions for their cause.

When all else fails, the homosexual movement has resorted to positive censorship in its attempts to keep views it considers obnoxious from the ears of the public. An example will suffice to show censorship as a political tool for enlisting the cooperation of hitherto unfriendly or neutral institutions in support of homosexuality. The following report appeared in *In Unity*, datelined Hartford: "The Gay Activist Alliance has convinced WOR-TV to edit and 'bleep' out anti-gay remarks made by Evangelist James Robinson (*sic*) on his weekly radio program. Robert Fennimore, general manager of WOR-TV, says 'If Robinson continues to attack homosexuals . . . he's going to be taken off the air.' "

This success in having a radio station exercise positive censorship of the remarks of a minister whose opinions are deemed contradictory to the interests and/or ideology of the homosexual movement makes such a station, in fact, part and parcel of the political efforts to impose the homosexual ideology. Several passages from the Bible attack homosexuality quite harshly. While modern revisionists have attributed meanings compatible with the homosexual ideology to these passages, the plain meaning of the translations that have been in use for hundreds of years and their traditional interpretation must be acknowledged as the views handed down by many generations. The logic of the general manager of WOR-TV would demand that a minister should be expelled from the air simply for reading the Scriptures!

In no way does everything in this chapter exhaust the political activities of the homosexual movement. Demonstrations and marches are also political activities. The act of "coming out" by a single homosexual is regarded by the movement as a political action. The homosexual movement is indeed political. Its aims are political, its methods are political, and its success would bring a political change to America the dimensions of which one cannot even begin to imagine.

CHAPTER THREE

The Homosexual Subculture

It is apparent even to a casual observer that in every sizable city—and even in many of our small communities—not only are there homosexuals, but many of these individuals have acquired certain social traits and developed patterns of behavior not directly connected to their sexual propensities. Of course, not all homosexuals—not even all those who have publicly "celebrated" their condition by "coming out"—exhibit all these traits and behaviors. But with many gays they serve to reinforce the homosexual's identity.

As a supplement to these traits and behaviors, a host of social institutions has developed which homosexuals utilize in "acting out" their homosexuality. These institutions include *bars* and *discos* where homosexuals drink, dance, relax, and find sex partners; homosexual *churches* and mainline-church-related groups, where they socialize while confirming their homosexuality from the ethical, theological, and cultural standpoints; *baths*, which are essentially places for engaging in one-to-one or group sex, either publicly or privately; *publications* in which homosexuals find information they need from their particular perspective, stimulation for their sexual fantasies in pornographic stores and photographs, and, when needed, the services of male prostitutes; *professional associations* where homosexuals meet their professional peers while

48   *Gays, AIDS and You*

advancing the interests of their cause; homosexual *prostitution* of young people who satisfy the desires of older individuals for an appropriate fee; and, finally, *homosexual "marriage"*, where homosexuals find companionship and mutual acceptability in the context of their sexual needs.

All these institutions, together with the various traits and behaviors, make up a peculiar subculture of American society. At this point the homosexual subculture is so vast and complex that it is virtually impossible to describe it all in detail. But it works together with the homosexual movement itself to provide the movement with its "flavor" and "distinctiveness," while receiving from the movement its perverse ideology. So in a sense, subculture and movement are two ways of looking at one and the same phenomenon.

Of course, the facets of the subculture are multiple. They range from the various institutions we've already mentioned to artistic and cultural events which are meant to advance the homosexual ideology while cementing the various components of the homosexual community. What follows are some examples of the subculture which will illustrate its chief characteristics:

OBJECTS AND SYMBOLS

There are literally hundreds of objects by which the homosexual can identify himself as a member of the subculture. A number of these objects are directly related to sexual practices, ranging from artificial electric masturbators—Accujacs—to such chemical products as butyl nitrite (poppers), a substance similar to the illegal drug amyl nitrite, which increases peripheral blood circulation and induces tachycardia, giving the user the illusion of a prolonged and more pleasurable orgasm. They include other items such as metal rings to be placed around the genitals; metal clips to cause pain in the male nipples; chains, whips, and leather straps with which sexual partners are ritually "punished"; dog collars and other gadgets designed to convey the feeling of inferiority and degradation on sexual partners; artificial male organs, and so forth.

Pornographic material is available at almost all prices and in a variety that would astonish—and appall—the inexperienced. There are inexpensive pornographic "novels," including some with illustrations, comic books, magazines, and tabloid newspapers featuring nude pictures, stories, and lewd advertisements. The only feature common to these publications seems to be the overwhelming preoccupation with sexuality. Homosexual printed matter is designed to satisfy the specific needs of the user. So there are items that concentrate on children having sex with one another, adults having sex with children, multi-ethnic and one-race publications, items which portray only individuals who have overdeveloped muscles using leather articles or motorcycles. In some cases the sexual activities depicted are of only one variety; other items depict a wide variety of sexual behavior. The sole purpose of these items is, of course, to provide sexual stimulation to the user.

Other objects which do not directly relate to sexual acts but which are indirectly—sometimes rather remotely—associated with homosexual practices include such items as greeting cards with homosexual themes (some with enormous genitals), naked attractive youths, or crude phrases descriptive of homosexual behavior; chocolates in the shapes of genitals; earrings for one ear, which many homosexuals use; sets of colored handkerchiefs which serve as a code by which homosexuals announce to each other their preferred practice (that is, each color corresponds to a certain sexual activity, while the side of the body where displayed indicates whether the person prefers to be active or passive); magnetic attachments for cars and refrigerators in the shape of individuals with over-developed genitals; "gay dolls" complete with fully stimulated genitals and a "closet"; purses, pocket books, change holders, book markers, key rings, and bumper-stickers—all centered around the theme of homosexuality.

Another powerful device which the homosexual movement has developed as the international symbol for homosexuality is the Greek letter lambda (λ). Since the early 1970s, λ has signified liberation for homosexuals, and it is now the acknowledged "logo" of the homosexual movement. It appears in publications and on bumper-stickers; ties with the lambda motiff are sold by mail and in homosexual shops; tie tacks, pendants, brooches, and other jewelry advertise the sexual interests of the wearer; six lambdas making up a "mogen David" constitute the symbol of Jewish homosexuality; Christian homosexual ministers have incorporated lambda in their sacred vestments and the vessels used for the celebration of the Eucharist. Lambda has indeed become the sign of homosexuality.

All these objects—from those closely connected with the most violent and degrading forms of sexual behavior to the lofty vestments by which homosexual ministers share with their congregation their own theological con-

viction that the homosexual condition is a God-given ave-
nue toward personal integration and sanctification—in
fact constitute powerful socializing agents for homosexuals who have chosen to affirm their sexual peculiarity. In
this process, they also become part of and help embody
the subculture of homosexuality as we know it today in
America.

HOMOSEXUAL BARS

Among all the social institutions within the homosexual
subculture, none has been more influential than the "gay
bar," of which there are several thousand nationwide.
(The *Gayellow Pages* lists 1,913 homosexual bars, and
clearly the total number is much higher.) These bars are
the meeting place for homosexuals. Indeed, from the ear-
liest times of the movement they have been at the center
of the effort to enshrine homosexuality as a legitimate
lifestyle.

Gay bars range from small "sleazy" places in dark and
dangerous alleys to plush establishments which compete
favorably with the best discotheques. Some bars cater to
a conventional-looking clientele. Other specialize in sa-
domasochists or transvestites. There are bars which pur-
posely attract young people, prostitutes who serve to attract older homosexuals who in turn purchase drinks for
youngsters while sexual deals are arranged. Printed
guides for traveling homosexuals or for newcomers usually specify what they can find at the various bars. This
includes the ethnic composition of the patrons, whether
the bar caters to homosexual males, females or a "mixed
crowd," whether heterosexuals are normally in attendance

TABLE 1

Homosexual Bars

Jurisdiction	Number	Jurisdiction	Number
Alabama	13	Montana	5
Alaska	4	Nebraska	10
Arizona	28	Nevada	10
Arkansas	8	New Hampshire	3
California	381	New Jersey	39
Colorado	16	New Mexico	7
Connecticut	15	New York	264
Delaware	5	North Carolina	19
District of Columbia	34	Ohio	65
Florida	130	Oklahoma	21
Georgia	32	Oregon	25
Hawaii	12	Pennsylvania	95
Idaho	2	Rhode Island	11
Illinois	82	South Carolina	8
Indiana	22	South Dakota	2
Iowa	9	Tennessee	26
Kansas	11	Texas	111
Kentucky	8	Utah	6
Louisiana	55	Vermont	2
Maine	13	Virginia	13
Maryland	22	Washington	33
Massachusetts	70	West Virginia	7
Michigan	48	Wisconsin	32
Minnesota	16	Wyoming	6
Mississippi	5	Puerto Rico	19
Missouri	26	Virgin Islands (US)	7
		Total	1913

SOURCE: *Gayellow Pages*, Renaissance House, New York, N.Y., 1981 edition.

or not, the availability of prostitutes or "rough trade" (that is, homosexuals who enjoy appearing violent or who actually behave violently) etc. Without the "gay bar," it would be impossible to conceive of the homosexual movement as it exists today. Homosexuals in fact trace the event which brought the movement into the open, the Stonewall riot, to an attempt by New York City police to curtail homosexual activity at a bar.

THE BATHS

Another institution that has been central to the homosexual subculture is the "gay bathhouse" or simply "the baths." While growing fear of AIDS among homosexuals has resulted in the closing down of many of these houses—due to lack of business—their role in the homosexual subculture is so central that a brief description is necessary to understand just what this subculture really looks like.

Although they are officially labeled "health clubs," the baths are really places where homosexuals find sexual partners. They make it possible for homosexuals to seek relief for their sexual urges without the need to establish personal relationships and to be burdened by the responsibilities these relationships imply. Baths provide their customers with a locker room for storing clothing or small cabins where homosexuals get together to have sex. There are also large rooms called "orgy rooms" or "mazes" where large numbers can congregate for group sex. The "better" baths also have screening rooms for the showing of pornographic films. In general there is little or no conversation except what is required for the establishment of a sexual liaison. The homosexuals simply wait, in poses that reflect their favorite sexual practices. In specialized establishments there are "dungeons" or "torture rooms" where homosexuals who wish to be degraded submit to sadists whose expertise is to inflict pain, punishment or humiliation. Special events to satisfy the specific needs of customers are also held. An example of such an event is the regular "slave auction" held at the Bulldog Baths in San Francisco on the second Wednesday of every month.

The degree of promiscuity in the baths defies the imagination of those not familiar with homosexuality. From the point of view of traditional values, they are probably some of the most destructive and degrading institutions in America today. There is no indication, however, that any of the homosexual organizations has opposed or in any way showed interest in counteracting the non-health-related effects of the baths. Indeed, it is only with the advent of AIDS that these baths have even become an issue within the homosexual community. Yet they constitute the antithesis of mental health, and ethically it is difficult if not impossible to justify on any moral grounds the impersonality and degradation these baths represent.

MUSIC AND THE ARTS

In addition to bars and baths, there are innumerable organizations and institutions which define and express the homosexual subculture. And it would be a mistake to assume that the only activities of liberated homosexuals within their community are to socialize, drink, and seek sexual partners in bars, or to participate in orgies at baths. In fact, there are many other activities within the homo-

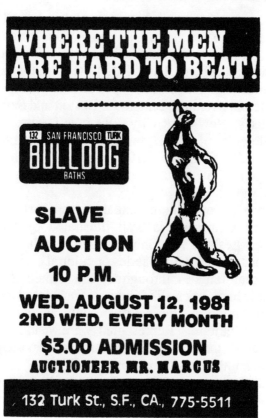

FIGURE 2.
SOURCE: *The* (San Francisco) *Sentinel,* August 7, 1981.

sexual community which have much in common with cultural activities of the rest of our society. However, it must be noted that there is an erotic component in most—if not all—activities identified as "gay."

One of the most viable, successful ventures of the homosexual movement is the San Francisco Gay Men's

Chorus, one of several homosexual bands and choral groups that exist in major U.S. cities. This group travels throughout the country, and is hosted by the most prestigious cultural centers. During its 1981 tour, for example, the Chorus was scheduled to perform at such places as the Dallas Convention Center, the Boston and Seattle Opera Houses, New York City's Beacon Theatre, and the national center of American culture, Washington D.C.'s Kennedy Center for the Performing Arts. While visiting Washington, the Chorus actually performed on the steps of the Capitol.

The production of homosexual works of art by the homosexual community is well illustrated by the Great American Lesbian Art Show, which was held in May 1980. This was actually a series of cultural events held by homosexual females throughout the United States. In large and small cities alike, homosexuals involved themselves in "honoring the creative contributions made by lesbians to culture." Represented were visual art, film, poetry, and other performances. It was reported by *In Unity* that 300 artists were represented in all.

Another case of homosexual art which had considerable public repercussions is the Gay Pride Sculpture in New York City. Created by George Segal, it constitutes a glorification of homosexuality, having the appropriate erotic undertones that characterize the homosexual subculture. The sculpture is made up of two homosexual couples, two males and two females. It became something of a cause celebre when attempts were made to install it in Sheridan Square, in the heart of Greenwich Village's homosexual neighborhood. The opposition of community groups was utilized by homosexual leaders as a political opportunity to raise the consciousness of their followers. The list of the project supporters provided by the Mariposa Foundation, funder of the project, comprises what can only be described as New York City's liberal establishment.

HOMOSEXUAL LITERATURE

The homosexual literature is crucial for the movement. Some of the most important homosexual professional organizations are the Discussion Group for Gay Studies in Language and Literature, an official body of the Modern Language Association, the Gay Caucus for the Modern Languages, and the Gay Task Force of the American Library Association. This is easy to understand, since literature is the ideal means for the transmittal of ideas. The ALA's Gay Task Force publishes and widely disseminates bibliographies centered on homosexuality from various viewpoints including religious, political, and sociological. These, in turn, are used by librarians, teachers, scholars, and activists to propagate the homosexual ideology while perpetuating the subculture itself. The Gay Caucus for the Modern Languages sponsors, among other activities, scholarly sessions with such titles as "Interpretive Problems in Nondeclared Lesbian Writers," and "Feminist Science Fiction: Utopian and Alternative Societies."

Bear in mind that one of the fundamental components of any subculture is its intelligentsia. The Gay Academic Union (GAU) is the focal point of the homosexual intelligentsia. Together with "gay achievers" and the "gay caucuses" of professional associations, the GAU promotes homosexuality from an intellectual platform. The by-laws of the Washington chapter of the Gay Academic Union state the following as the purpose of the organization: "The Gay Academic Union is a voluntary organization of individuals who have a scholarly interest in homosexuality and the gay/lesbian subculture. The purpose of the organization is to increase the knowledge of the members, to provide opportunities for professional and social contacts, and to serve as a resource for the gay community."

The GAU sponsors programs which, in the long run, are bound to result in the strengthening of the homosexual subculture. Its award program includes the granting of Literary, Fine Arts, and the Evelyn Hooker Research awards. Such activities as a lecture on homosexuals' participation in World War II, Lesbian History, and Sexual Politics in the '80s indicate the existence of the intellectual component of the homosexual subculture.

In sum, it would be accurate to describe the homosexual subculture as a complex web of interlocking organizations and institutions. They "resocialize" their members, and provide them with political, social, psychological, and at times even economic support. Once a person becomes involved in this subculture, he or she has little reason to leave it; immersion in the subculture may become total. Some of the elements in this subculture even facilitate the relief from sexual needs which undoubtedly assail every homosexual.

Strange as it may appear, becoming a full-fledged member of the homosexual subculture entails centering one's life on one's sexual peculiarities. It constitutes an ever-stronger bonding of the homosexual to others like himself, thus decreasing the individual's freedom even as it provides him with a sense of liberation. From a traditional point of view, this is no liberation at all, but rather enslavement to an all-consuming passion. In short, "gay liberation" is not merely the acquisition of social and political privileges as a "legitimate minority," but a freeing of the homosexual to seek the complete satisfaction of his sexual appetites without the restrictions which children, family responsibility, and the tenets of the Judeo-Christian ethic impose on heterosexuals.

In this way, the homosexual subculture is solidly anchored in the psychosexual needs of its members which, in turn, it heightens. The more deeply the homosexual participates in "his" subculture, the stronger is his condition. Conversely, the deeper the homosexuality, the stronger the subculture in which he exists.

There are two aspects of the homosexual subculture which, although not related to each other, reflect the nature of the subculture and its interaction with American society. On the one hand, the possibility that homosexuality is an illness and thus a sexual disorder makes the subculture unique. This is especially true when you consider that homosexuality involves the will and human consciousness—that is, it is not just a physical condition. There are certain other illnesses which, while not physically the result of the homosexual condition, are clearly related to the practice of homosexuality. And since many of these illnesses are infectious, and their treatment at times uses vast amount of public money, their existence is important for our entire society.

On the other hand, one of the factors which has created the homosexual subculture—and a tool widely used by the movement to accomplish its objectives—is language. To truly understand this subculture we need to look at this a bit more closely.

LANGUAGE AND THE HOMOSEXUAL SUBCULTURE

A visit to any homosexual bookstore reveals the existence of a number of glossaries, some of them quite extensive, which provide the uninitiated with thousands of words by which homosexuals describe themselves, the world, and especially their sexual activities. The appendices of modern books on homosexuality often provide glossaries so that readers can made sense of the quotes from homosexuals. In short, there is no question but that the homosexual subculture has developed what amounts to its own language. Moreover, this language has created a perception of homosexuality that is social and political by its nature. Thus to be homosexual is a political act, an affirmation of power. Not surprisingly, homosexual organizations try to sensitize their members to the power of language. During the 1979 convention of the National Council of Teachers of English, the homosexual caucus within this organization sponsored a program entitled "Panel on the language of heterosexism." Aside from two homosexual poetry readings, this was their only substantive activity at the convention.

One of the most important contributions of the homosexual movement to contemporary English usage is the word "gay." This key word is utilized to create the sexual class consciousness of members of the movement, to create the social environment in which new members of the subculture feel welcome, supported, and proud by providing members with pride and self-acceptance. "Gay" is used to distinguish the person who merely feels sexually attracted to members of his or her own sex from those who also *celebrate* this attraction, define this attraction as "good," and identify those who suffer from this attraction with others who are like them. In addition, "gay" serves to create and point to the supportive environment and the services a homosexual can find in bars, baths, churches, bookstores, health clinics, beauty parlors, radio programs, and restaurants.

In short, within the homosexual subculture "gay" is a magical word that has a creative power of its own. In the minds and perceptions of its users, it is the key indicator for today's liberated homosexual that he has nothing to fear from that to which he is pegged. He is "gay," "all-gay," and anything "gay" is part of him.

The sociopolitical significance of "gay" is thus apparent. If anything, the homosexual movement needs its acceptance as a matter of sheer survival. Naturally, should "gay" cease to be used, many people would still be attracted to members of their own sex, homosexuality would still be practiced, and some parts of the subculture would still be fully in place. *In accepting without any resistance the use of "gay," American society and government have, in fact, bought into the homosexual movement. By the same token, profamily and other traditional value-oriented activists can wage a most effective campaign against homosexuality simply by insisting on the abolition of "gay" (in its prohomosexual sense) as an accepted word.*

HOMOSEXUAL LANGUAGE IN RELIGION

Today in America, the homosexual and feminist movements have joined forces to provoke a change in the language by which religion is fashioned and expressed. The proposed change consists in the usage of inclusive or non-sexist language, wherein all references to God or persons in general by the use of "masculine" words is eliminated. One of the obvious and most damaging effects of this change is to blur the distinction between genders and the attribution of specific roles according to gender. Naturally, anything that contributes to the blurring of gender-related distinctions is supported by the homosexual movement.

For example, during the Seventh General Conference of the Universal Fellowship of Metropolitan Community Churches (UFMCC) in Washington, D.C. in 1976, the Task Force on Women presented the following resolution:

> Resolved that UFMCC, at this General Conference, reaffirming the recommendation of the UFMCC 1975 General Conference, direct its member churches to continue to change the language used during worship services (including hymns, liturgy, scripture and sermons) and that each church use inclusive (nonsexist) language therein, as informed by guidelines supplied by the Task Force on Women and the Commission on Faith Fellowship and Orders.

Two women leaders of the UFMCC, Marge Rogona and Jennie Bull, have, the group reported, "put together an excellent manual called 'De-Sexing Your Local Hymnal,' which provides a guide to language problems in over 700 of our favorite hymns."

The ultimate source of religious language in America is the Bible; thus the UFMCC announced (with obvious glee) the attempts of the National Council of Churches (NCC) to reinterpret the Scriptures according to the dictates of the homosexual and feminist movements:

The National Council of Churches' task force on biblical translation is recommending that the NCC prepare a new lectionary with an emphasis on inclusive and nonsexist language. The task force also suggested to the RSV Bible Committee, who is presently working on an updated version to be published in the mid–1980s, that they consider studying the possibility of a separate inclusive language New Testament building on the new lectionary.

The task force has recommended using the word "children" for "sons" and "ancestors" for "patriarchs."

In fact, the incorporation of inclusive language in the Bible or other sacred writing amounts to a reinterpretation of the text. By imposing the newly found categories on the original language, the message intended by the authors is twisted to serve the ideological—and thus political—aims of homosexuals and feminists alike. The parallel passages in Table 2 will allow the reader to see the effect of using inclusive language in reinterpreting the Scriptures.

There is no doubt that the homosexual subculture has not only developed a peculiar language, but that this language is structured and functions in a manner designed to satisfy the needs of the homosexual movement and its members. Their needs are not "identificational" but political. And if our discussion of the language of the homosexual subculture is not sufficient to make the point, even a cursory examination of an official glossary prepared by the State of California shows the ideological function of the language of homosexuality. Practically every element of the homosexual ideology is enshrined in this document. Produced under the direction of the Sexual Orientation Project of the State Personnel Board, and purport-

TABLE 2

Passage	King James Version of the Bible	Inclusive Language
Mark 14:62	And Jesus said, "I am; and ye shall see the Son of man sitting on the right hand of power, and coming in the clouds of heaven."	Then Jesus said, "I am. And you will see Humanity's Child sitting at the right hand of power, and coming with the clouds of heaven."
Mark 14:36	And he said, "Abba, Father, all things are possible unto thee; take away this cup from me: nevertheless not what I will, but what thou wilt."	And he said, "Holy source of my being, all things are possible to you; remove this cup from me. Yet, not what I desire, but what you will."
John 1:51	And he saith unto him, "Verily, verily, I say unto you, hereafter ye shall see heaven open, and the angels of God ascending and descending upon the Son of man."	And Jesus continued, "Thus truly I tell you, you will see heaven opened, and the angels of God going up and coming down upon the Child of Humanity.

ing to represent "the current state of social scientific research in the area of sexual orientation," the glossary is in fact a political tool for the promotion of the homosexual ideology within the California State government.

The language of the homosexual subculture is not just a means of communication. It is fundamentally a political tool by which the movement seeks to increase its political power, impose its ideology, and thus provoke a fundamental change in our thought and social practice. Although it would be naive to assume that if this language should cease to be used the homosexual movement would disappear immediately, it is probable that a well-organized campaign within schools, professional and religious bodies, economic institutions, and the media would contribute, by exposing the true character of the homosexual language, to a substantial check on the acceptance of the homosexual ideology. Such a move would be fiercely resisted, since it would spell the intellectual demise of the homosexual subculture.

Should the homosexual language and ideology prevail, our society would have no way of speaking—or thinking—in traditional terms. Conversely, should the profamily forces prevail, homosexual acts would come to be viewed as a manifestation of sinfulness, an illness, or a potential and/or actual source of crime. In any case, it would be seen as a form of psychosocial disruption. Once it was viewed this way—even by the homosexuals themselves—the movement would cease to exist.

CHAPTER FOUR

The Homosexual Ideology

Acceptance of the homosexual ideology in America would bring about a fundamental, revolutionary change in our society. We would see an *immediate rejection* of such fundamental values as: the traditional distinction between male and female; the character of the traditional American family; the ability of parents to be the main agents in the raising of their children; the tenets of religion and rational ethics in the area of human sexuality; the prohibition of prostitution, pornography, incest, free sex, adult/child sexual relationships, child pornography, and so forth.

David Thorstad, a spokesman for the North American Man/Boy Love Association, has articulated an ideology of homosexuality which includes these components:

1. *Sex.* In all its forms, sex is good so long as it is consensual. Specifically, homosexuality is good for those who practice it:

> NAMBLA takes the view that sex is good, that homosexuality is good not only for adults, but for young people as well. We support all consensual sexual relationships regardless of age. As long as the relationship is mutually pleasurable, and no one's right are violated, sex should be no one else's business.

2. *Children's Liberation.* The concept of "liberation" is central to the homosexual ideology. For the homosexual

movement, liberation means the ability of all homosexuals and their partners to be free of all external and internal constraints in the pursuit of sexual pleasure. According to NAMBLA:

> Sexual liberation cannot be achieved without the liberation of children. This means many things. Children need to gain control over their lives, a control which they are denied on all sides. They need to break the yoke of "protection" which alienates them from themselves, a "protection" imposed on them by adults—their family, the schools, the state, and prevailing sexual and social mores.

3. *Motherhood.* At the center of the homosexual ideology seems to be the need or desire to challenge the traditional family centered on a loving relationship between a man and a woman for the purpose of begetting children. Biologically, of course, homosexual activities are nonproductive. Thus a homosexual "family" stands out in sharp contrast to the traditional family. NAMBLA, which represents the ideological edge of the homosexual movement, directly challenges the very concept of the traditional family:

> With the decline of the extended family and traditional church influence, the state has increased its investment in maintaining a preferred family structure, i.e., male-dominated, heterosexual, nuclear variety . . . The greatest threat to this . . . repressive system is presented by sexual and affectionate personal relations outside the approved mode. Specifically, this means the freedom of those over whom the state still has greatest control (minors) and those with whom they would create their own lives . . . Mothering the young is a role imposed on women, frequently against their will.

4. *Age of Consent.* Central to the homosexual ideology is the idea that all people should decide everything for themselves—without regard to tradition or "normal" behavior patterns. So while moral limitations have traditionally been accepted as enhancing individual freedom, the homosexual movement separates the sexual practices of consenting partners from moral considerations. This is crucial for NAMBLA:

> There is no age at which a person becomes capable of consenting to sex. The age of sexual consent is just one of many ways in which adults impose their system of control on children . . . The state is the enemy of freedom, not its guarantor. The best evidence against the argument that children cannot consent to sex, including with adults, is the fact that millions do it anyway.

To support its peculiar ideology, the homosexual movement pours a great deal of effort into arguing about what homosexuality is *not*. More precisely, the movement insists that homosexuality is not a matter of choice, and that it is not changeable. Let's take a closer look at these two (flawed) arguments:

HOMOSEXUALITY IS NOT A MATTER OF CHOICE

An almost universal theme within the homosexual movement is the idea that homosexuals are in no way responsible for being the way they are. In the process of growing up, homosexual writers assert, a person "discovers" that he is homosexual. So the acquisition of a "homosexual consciousness" is seen as a process of self-discovery and maturation, rather than as involving a choice on the part of the homosexual. Of course, this statement is ideological rather than scientific in nature—that is, it has been formulated for the explicit purpose of serving the goals and objectives of the homosexual movement.

This is a particularly important question for the homosexual movement. If it could be shown that homosexuality has nothing to do with choice, the movement would be able to count on the support of many heterosexuals who would have come to believe that it is unavoidable.

The homosexual movement has been trying for years to make prohomosexual legislation conform to this ideological tenet. For example, Andy Humm, a New York City homosexual leader, speaking about the 1981 version of the New York City homosexual rights bill, said this:

> What makes this bill new is a simplification of language. The bill which has been defeated for ten years adds the category of "sexual orientation" to the list of bases on which one may not discriminate, and defines sexual orientation as "the choice of sexual orientation according to gender." This definition is thought to be limiting, inaccurate, and uninstructive. It introduces the concept of choice when we are trying to establish sexual orientation as an innate part of human personality. Thus, the definition will be dropped. . . .

A similar change was introduced in the 1979 Weiss-Waxman prohomosexual bill (H.R. 2074). The participation of the homosexual leadership in the drafting of this bill and the incorporation of the homosexual ideology in its language and intent are evident:

> . . . Major changes have been made in the bill, after consultation between the UFMCC Washington Office, the Gay Rights National Lobby, other Gay organizations, and Mem-

bers of Congress and their aides. First, the old term "affec-
tional or sexual preference," has been changed to "affec-
tional or sexual orientation." The reason for this is that it
was felt "orientation" best expresses the nature of human
sexuality, while "preference" raises the possibility that we
believe sexuality is a matter of choice.

HOMOSEXUALITY IS NOT CHANGEABLE

As we have pointed out, the unchangeability of the homosexual condition is also a central ideological tenet of
the movement. Thus not only is the individual "locked"
into being a homosexual, but attempts to change him are
themselves immoral. It is not surprising that this should
be so central a theme to the homosexual ideology: a denial
of the possibility of change implies for homosexual leaders the responsibility of the rest of society to accept homosexuality as normal. Moreover, legally it becomes impossible to demand that an individual attempt to change a
condition. And since change is impossible, and the individual is not responsible for his condition (the homosexual leaders contend), no legal or moral guilt can be im-
puted.

This issue has practical consequence of great importance for the homosexual movement. In the case of James
Gaylord, a homosexual teacher who admitted his condition to his principal, the Washington Supreme Court re-
fused to force his readmission as a teacher on the basis—
among others—that he "desired no change and has sought
no psychiatric help" to change his sexual orientation,
therefore, "He had made a voluntary choice for which he
must be held morally responsible." It is thus vital for ho-

mosexuals to assert that they cannot change, lest they be forced to undergo such a conversion.

Of course, the perception that homosexuality is unchangeable is *not* universally accepted outside the homosexual movement. Such traditional psychotherapists as Edmund Bergler and Irving Bieber believe that homosexuality is indeed changeable. According to Bieber, out of seventy-two patients, 38 percent had become heterosexuals or bisexuals (19 percent each) and 27 percent had shifted from homosexuality and bisexuality to exclusively heterosexuality. The process is long and tedious, sometimes requiring over 350 hours of therapy. Similarly, sex therapists William H. Masters and Virginia Johnson have indicated, on the basis of a 15-year study on more than 300 male and female homosexuals, that they were successful in helping two-thirds of the 54 men and 13 women who indicated a desire to become heterosexual.

To further support its ideology, the homosexual movement has developed three separate but related themes:

—"Coming Out" is a desirable action.
—Homosexuality in itself has no moral implications.
—Homophobia is an undesirable, indeed repugnant, condition.

These three themes are central to the homosexual ideology. They provide a set of guideposts for homosexuals themselves. And, more importantly, they provide political ammunition for use against those who oppose the spread of the homosexual ideology. Let us look at each theme more closely, to see how it supports the homosexual ideology and helps the movement to fulfill its political agenda.

'COMING OUT' IS A DESIRABLE ACTION

In the homosexual movement, coming to terms with the homosexual condition requires undergoing a process called "coming out," which is not unlike a religious conversion. It is important to understand that coming out is not just becoming aware that one is homosexual and accepting this as a fact. Anyone with a modicum of psychic stability, on realizing that he is a homosexual, will come to accept that he is affected by this condition. Indeed, the precondition for any effort to change from homosexual to heterosexual or celibate homosexual is the acceptance that homosexuality is present. Coming out (a shortened version of "coming out of the closet") implies an appreciation and acceptance that homosexuality is good. And the implication of such an acceptance is nothing less than a rejoicing in the homosexual condition, hence the word "gay" by which "liberated" or "out" homosexuals describe their sexuality. It also demands the communication of this feeling and self-knowledge to others. Hence Adam DeBaugh says that "coming out is a bit of verbal shorthand for the concept of coming out of the closet. It means, for most gay people, accepting, celebrating, and sharing the truth about who they are sexually."

Coming out is not a singular event, although at times a homosexual comes out *to* one or another person. In some instances, telling significant others in his life—parents, teachers, a trusted friend or minister—is spoken of as a homosexual's coming out. However, coming out is best described as a *process* by which a homosexual becomes a "fully actualized person." In the final analysis we can say that a homosexual never stops "coming out," since new levels of self-awareness are always possible, and new forms of discrimination always remain to be conquered.

Coming out is a progressive form of identification with the homosexual condition, a continuing and increasing commitment to homosexuality itself as a positive and creative thing. By coming out, the homosexual creates around himself a web of relationships and situations from which he finds it virtually impossible to break free. The initial perception that homosexuality is unchangeable is strengthened when the person brands himself as "different" on account of his sexual proclivities. Moreover, the people to whom the homosexual comes out also begin to perceive the homosexual not only as someone who *now* likes people of his own sex, but as someone who cannot help but feel this way and who acts on his feelings in the practice of homosexuality. The homosexual, while coming out, might acquire one or more sexual partners who are introduced to others as "lovers." In cases where the homosexual becomes a member of a homosexually oriented church, or a homosexual group within one of the established churches, the partners might have undergone the rite of "holy gay union," which in their view is similar to marriage.

For the movement, the importance of homosexuals coming out lies precisely in the effect this process has in raising the consciousness of the homosexual. In a sense, it is coming out that makes a homosexual part of the movement. The political consequences of coming out are clear. Indeed, DeBaugh has identified political and communal action as the last step in the process: "The last step is coming out politically. When we begin to understand the depth of our oppression as gay people, and we begin to act on that understanding, we are coming out in political ways."

This means lobbying Congress and other legislative bodies on behalf of homosexuality, being willing to serve as plaintiff in court cases, pressuring the administrative and executive branches of government, contacting business and private organizations on behalf of the movement, and similar activities. This is what, in fact, constitutes the homosexual movement. *For without coming out, there would be no movement. Homosexuals who come out transcend their individuality; while remaining homosexual and actively following up their sexual inclinations, their political devotion to their community becomes paramount in their lives.*

HOMOSEXUALITY IN ITSELF HAS NO MORAL IMPLICATIONS

Morality is not only an expression of the ethical value of human behavior and social structures, but one of the strongest forces in sharing and controlling them. When homosexuality is seen as having ethical connotations, these can be used to curb the sexual behavior of homosexuals. So much of the movement's support has its roots in the ability to satisfy (or justify the satisfaction of) the needs of its members—including the perceived need to have sexual relations with persons of the same sex—that an ideological statement that denies the attachment of any ethical value to homosexuality itself must logically be part of the movement's belief system.

This does not mean that homosexuals will affirm ethi-

cal indifference to any and every action in the practice of
their sexual activity. Rather, it means that homosexuality
in itself has no ethical connotations. Those homosexuals
who profess to be religious, and who have integrated their
"gay is good" ideology with their sexual practices and
religious beliefs, will, in fact, affirm that homosexual actions are morally good. However, there is never the implication that homosexuality has moral significance. The
ethics of the homosexual action are seen as coming from
the intention of the homosexuals rather than from the actions themselves.

In short, sexual preference is to be divorced from morality. Ideologically, this divorce is a very convenient device since it precludes the possibility of evaluating homosexual behavior from an ethical point of view. From a
financial point of view, homosexual behavior may be
quite lucrative—for example, for male prostitutes, homosexual bar and bath owners, manufacturers of homosexual paraphernalia, and the pornography industry. From
a hedonistic point of view, homosexual behavior is pleasurable.

Psychologically, *once values are removed from the
scene*, homosexual behavior can be advocated as helpful
in providing homosexuals with self-identification. Politically, homosexuality is said to be an asset, since the "homosexual community" constitutes a powerful voting bloc.
It is the question of morality that remains a barrier for
homosexuals as individuals and for the movement as a
social force. Thus the movement clears the way toward
"total sexual freedom" by declaring that homosexuality
and morality are, in reality, unrelated items.

HOMOPHOBIA IS AN UNDESIRABLE CONDITION

One of the commonest terms in the homosexual literature is "homophobia." This newly coined word, always used in a negative context, constitutes the counterpart of "gay." All that has been said positively about "gay" is repeated, in a negative way, about "homophobia." If being "gay" is the condition of accepting and affirming joyfully the fact that one is a homosexual, "homophobia" means the rejection of such a condition. In its need to promote the value of homosexuality, the movement thus considers homophobia as a most undesirable condition. It is spoken of as an illness that has to be cured, a form of discrimination that has to be obliterated and, in the religious context, a sin that must be forgiven.

The simplest and most concise definition of homophobia is given by Ralph Blair, the psychotherapist director of the Homosexual Community Counseling Center and president of Evangelicals Concerned (a prohomosexual religious group). According to Blair, "homophobia is an expression of fear of homosexuality."

To the theoreticians of the homosexual movement, homophobia refers not only to societal values and preconceptions among heterosexuals, but also to individual feelings and deeply ingrained personality structures. Thus, the concept of homophobia enables the homosexual movement to link arms with other "liberation movements" not only in America but throughout the world. Joan Clark, fired in the late 1970s from the staff of the Women's Division, Board of Global Ministries of the United Methodist Church after she came out as a female homosexual, has clearly linked the "antihomophobia" struggle with other aspects of liberation theology (the reinterpretation of Christianity in Marxist categories). In an article that appeared in *Integrity Forum*, the official publication of Episcopalian homosexuals, she asserts: "I will focus on the struggle to eliminate homophobia as a commitment to justice with the depth, power, and intertwining of issues that characterize other liberation struggles, i.e., those to eliminate racism, sexism, classism, and imperialism."

One indication of just how seriously the homosexual movement depends on the notion of homophobia to pursue its ideology can bee seen from an address by Ralph Blair to the Strategy Conference on Homophobia in the Churches. In his address, Dr. Blair prescribed a strategy to combat the problems and indicated pitfalls to be avoided. Table 3, based on Blair's address, summarizes his approach.

It is interesting to note that Marxist homosexuals attribute homophobia to the rise of private property. In their bizarre interpretation the rejection of homosexuality is also linked with its nonprocreative nature. Thus, according to one Marxist homosexual group, "Homosexual relations did not produce children. This fact by itself is enough to account for the fact that homosexuality came to be disparaged at the same time that private wealth began to be coveted."

The elimination of homophobia is an important goal of the homosexual movement, and the struggle against this condition is being waged on a continuing basis. As a matter of fact, one could conceive of the movement itself as a gigantic effort to end homophobia, thus allowing homosexuals to give free rein to their desires, however bizarre they would have been considered under "homophobic" conditions.

We have already seen some of the strategies Dr. Ralph

Blair has prescribed against homophobia. New Ways Ministry a Catholic pro-homosexual organization, utilizes an "Index of Attitudes Toward Homosexual People" which enables those who use it to confront their own feelings toward homosexuality and thus have the opportunity to modify these feelings. The index is in the form of twenty-five questions scored on a five-point scale. The subject is confronted with twelve "prohomosexual" statements such as "I would feel comfortable if a member of my own sex made an advance toward me," and "if a member of my sex made an advance toward me I would feel flattered," and thirteen anti-homosexual statements such as "I would feel uncomfortable if I learned that my spouse or partner was attracted to members of his/her own sex," and "I would feel disappointed if I learned that my child was homosexual." Such expressions of self-disclosure are bound to bring a confrontation with tradition-minded individuals who have otherwise accepted—intellectually only—the homosexual ideology, or who are struggling with the issue. As a result of this value conflict, and under the pressure of the "progressive" attitude that constitutes the framework in which the homosexual ideology is normally presented, the individual is forced to give up his homophobia and embrace the homosexual ideology.

While homosexual organizations will seldom, if ever, describe themselves as revolutionary, a clear understanding of the movement's nature and of some statements made by homosexual leaders shows that this is indeed the case. American society has traditionally been conservative, and throughout the 1970s and into the 1980s public sentiment has grown consistently more so. So it would be disruptive for the homosexual movement to proclaim its revolutionary nature openly; its leaders rarely mention it.

The word "revolutionary" is used here in two senses,

TABLE 3

"Homophobia": Alleged Sources and Solutions Proposed

Source of Homophobia	Problem Statement	Prescribed Strategy	Pitfalls to be avoided
1) The Bible and Theology	*The Bible and biblical theology speak against homosexuality.* This is a proposition which some people use "to justify a priori sentiments, including homophobia." (p. 9)	"Patiently [to] present as clear an opportunity as possible to take the Bible seriously and to assist any who would wish to know better what the Bible does and does not say." (p. 10)	Calling "homophobes" those who sincerely believe that the Bible speaks against homosexuality. (p. 10)
2) Treatment and "Deliverance" Promises	*Homosexuality is sinful.* . . . [I]f only homosexuals would 'get saved' they would be 'delivered' from homosexuality. This is not possible." (p. 11)	"To assist them—i.e., the homophobes—to realize that there is no cure for what is not a disease and there is no healing or deliverance from that which is not a spiritual affliction. (p. 12)	"Make fun of them and pretend that they constitute a small minority of backwater fundamentalists." (p. 11)
3) Prejudice	"Another way in which Christians might tend to be what we might call homophobic . . . is by way of preconceived notions of what homosexuality is." (p. 12)	Counter the thinking that all homosexuals are leftists, promiscuous, pro-abortion, etc. (p. 13)	None indicated.

4) Civil Religion and Americanism	"The following statement from Adolph Hitler is accepted throughout the Bible Belt and in other segments of American Christianity: 'We just seek firmly to protect Christianity as the basis of our entire morality, and the family as the nucleus of the life of our people.'" (p. 13)	Speak up when "politics or neurotic excesses" are presented as "homosexuality." (p. 15)	Knee-jerk reaction that results in the "gay community" speaking with one voice. (p. 15)
5) Defense Mechanism	"Some people use homosexuals and the gay rights issues, etc. to defend themselves against their own deep sense of guilt, inadequacy, and insecurity." (p. 16)	Assess whether one is dealing with a person who is "honestly misinformed" or is using "homophobia as a defense mechanism." Respond accordingly. If the homophobic person is insecure or feels inferior, provide the required reassurance. (p. 16)	Engage the homophobe in strenuous arguments in which the prohomosexual party presents very powerful reasons to support his position (pp. 16 and 18)

NOTE: All page numbers from Blair, *Homophobia in the Churches*.

and the homosexual ideology qualifies under both of them. On the one hand, revolutionary can mean the inversion of a way of thinking. Should the homosexual ideology become the dominant force in American society, a change of such magnitude would become inevitable. Revolutionary also means an identification with one or more principles held by other radical organizations which advocate total changes in our social, economic, or political structures outside our traditional constitutional framework. This identification exists across the board among homosexual leaders and organizations. In both instances, the revolutionary nature of the homosexual movement makes it a political phenomenon. In being revolutionary, the movement satisfies not only its own needs but the needs of its members, who must perceive that the goals and activities of the movement will predictably create the social and political conditions in which they will be free to engage in their favorite sexual practices.

It was during the 1960s that the homosexual movement took on its revolutionary character. More recently, the more extreme leftist rhetoric of the movement has been largely abandoned, at least by some leaders. However, as we have already seen, the homosexual organization of the Episcopal Church listed typically radical issues as some of the movement's own issues. And a minister of the pro-homosexual Metropolitan Community Church identified with sexism—against which the homosexual movement stands—typically leftist issues:

> People must deal with the chains that destroy us. Wrapped up in this sexist issue is the key to freedom. Contained within the bondage of sexism is racism and classism, homophobia, and the rape and plunder of our earth.

In sum, then, it is clear that the homosexual movement has a consistent and highly developed ideology. Not all homosexuals, not even all those who have come out, fully share every principle we have presented here. These principles, however, do satisfy the needs of the movement and its members. They serve to frame the issues of importance to the movement, which are political by nature. Like all ideologies, the homosexual ideology is neither scientific nor objective. Its statements are "working principles" designed to increase the ability of liberated homosexuals to modify their social environment for their own benefit. Any denial of these principles, especially when such denial is enshrined in laws or public policy, is bound to elicit a strong and perhaps violent reaction by the homosexual movement.

However, the preservation of traditional society and the values that most Americans cherish requires the denial of the homosexual ideology. While it is impossible to predict whether or not the homosexual movement will prevail, it is obvious that should this movement prevail in America, the nation we have known would cease to exist.

CHAPTER FIVE

Homosexuality and Religion

It is crucial to understand how important religion is—and
the support of religious institutions—to the homosexual
movement. And it is crucial to understand how exten-
sively the homosexual movement has already infiltrated
our country's mainline churches.

Bear in mind that organized religion is not only the
social institution to which the greatest number of people
belong voluntarily, but also the single most influential
factor in the evaluation of behavior. As individuals, even
those who do not formally belong to a church or attend
religious services obtain much guidance from religious
institutions in forming their consciences. Moreover, a religion provides its adherents with precise rules which enable them to measure the ethical qualities of their personal
behavior. In a sense, religion structures reality for the
individual and categorizes the nature and value of his relationships.

The presence of religious organizations in any country
affects individuals not only as believers, but also as members of society. In a society such as the United States,
where religion played such a preeminent role in the foundation of the nation itself, and where there is a rather
weak antireligious tradition, religious organizations have
an especially fundamental role. It is true that forces representative of secular humanism (embodied by such insti-

tutions as Planned Parenthood Federation, the American Civil Liberties Union, Americans for Democratic Action, and others) have tried to undermine the degree to which religion is an accepted factor in American life. In a formal sense they have succeeded to a great extent, inasmuch as there has been a rejection of customs and practices which, having their roots in religion, contributed to the growth of the religious dimension in Americans, although they were in themselves secular and rational in nature. It is indeed ironic that secular humanist institutions are so bent on destroying the very foundations of Western Civilization which has enabled them to exist!

There is no question that the main stumbling block in the theoretical and practical acceptance of homosexuality by American society has been traditional religion. This has been perfectly understood by the leadership of the homosexual movement. For many years systematic efforts to utilize religion in support of homosexuality have been implemented not only by the founding of religious organizations which cater almost exclusively to homosexuals while purporting to justify their sexual propensities and activities, but also by the establishment of organizations within other religious institutions for the purpose of using them for the promotion of the homosexual ideology.

The supreme importance of gaining the support of the churches—or at least neutralizing them—is widely acknowledged by homosexual leaders. At a Washington meeting of Friends for Lesbian and Gay Concerns (FLGC), a Quaker organization, concern was expressed over the apparent lack of support for homosexuality from the Friends Committee on National Legislation, an important body within the denomination. The meeting was attended by one Steve Endean, director of Gay Rights National Lobby, who apparently prodded the attendees to enlist the collaboration of their church in the homosexual cause. Endean, according to the official newsletter of FLGC, "outlined for us the significance that such a position of support from FCNL would have on national legislators and other church lobby groups—some of which would be less timid about supporting gay rights if the Friends (FCNL) were doing so. The support of these church lobbies would be important in offsetting the negativism from the Christian right led by the Christian Voice, the new lobby set up to wage their war against us." The clear implication is that homosexual Quakers should use their resources to set their religious organizations against another—more traditional—Christian group and support the homosexual movement.

The homosexual ideology presents such a radical departure from traditional religious teaching—to the point of contradicting it—that it has become necessary for the religious apologists of homosexuality to introduce wholly new principles that enable a total rejection of the traditional teachings while keeping all the appearances and control mechanisms of religion intact. Thus the new dogma of homosexuality can be enshrined. The principles in question are *moral relativism* and *situation ethics*, both of which fully satisfy the requirement that the practice of homosexuality be acceptable. A good example of the use of moral relativism is the testimony in favor of prohomosexual legislation offered by the Reverend Cecil Williams at a Congressional hearing where the following exchange took place:

> Mr. Stephens: Let me ask questions of Reverend Williams. I think it unfortunate that you have experienced the prejudice and discrimination that you have and that people have been prejudiced to you in the name of the Scriptures. I, too, think it is abhorrent. But one thing which concerns me is

the distinction between the behavior of people and what Scripture teaches. Are there certain moral absolutes which don't change from era to era?

Reverend Williams: There are no absolutes. All absolutes have to be looked at, criticized, reinterpreted, revised. That is why you have revised versions of the Bible. It is to reestablish, redirect, make relevant, the word (*sic*) in different circumstances. That is merely one way of looking at it. There are no absolutes that should not and cannot be reinterpreted and redefined as well as to create different responses for the times during which people live.

This is no less than a religious revolution. Whereas traditional religion would use the Bible as a guide, we see here the Bible as the maidservant of the trends of the times. In other words, the Bible is placed at the service of the homosexual ideology. Any objective basis for religion disappears, sacrificed at the altar of the individual's sexual needs, however bizarre. The preoccupation of many in the homosexual movement with religion and Biblical teaching, the very need to reject traditional Biblical morality, bears witness to the importance attached to these teachings.

In the final analysis, the key question is whether religious mechanisms can significantly influence the homosexual's need to fulfill his sexual desires either alone or with one or more partners. Thus the claim of religion to arrest or even to reverse homosexuality is a challenge of incalculable magnitude to the homosexual movement. It is not surprising that the movement responded so virulently to an article whose very title, "Homosexuals CAN Change," indicated the thesis that with God's help a person can cease to be an active homosexual. Such a claim *must* be neutralized, for if it were to be accepted there would be no reason for people to continue the practice of homosexuality. All homosexual claims of "goodness" or "inevitability" would have to be rejected. The homosexual movement would indeed come to a screeching halt.

Thus religion is a threat to the homosexual movement. Alas, the present state of flux in American society, and the progressive secularization of certain religious organizations, have made some of these institutions easy prey for the well-organized efforts of the homosexual movement. Its leaders have not only acknowledged the importance of this support, they use it prominently. The National Gay Task Force, for example, publishes a packet of documentation issued by representatives of groups as diverse as the Union of American Hebrew Congregations and the General Convention of the Episcopal Church, showing various degrees of support for the homosexual movement. This support is then used by the movement's leadership to support it goals. The following quote taken from a letter from the executive director of the Gay Rights National Lobby to *The Washington Star* in support of pro-homosexual legislation is a good example of how this religious support is used:

> Many religious leaders, organizations and denominations, including the National Council of Churches, the National Federation of Priests' Councils [a Chicago-based Roman Catholic organization] and the Union of American Hebrew Congregations, have understood the distinction between support for civil rights legislation for gay people and any moral judgments about homosexuality. They do agree that discrimination is wrong and immoral.

One result of the homosexual movement's recognition of the importance of religion in approving their ideology in America is the targeting of religious institutions for a prohomosexual "public education" campaign by the National Gay Task Force. This campaign has as its goal "to make a positive impact on the perceptions of lesbians and gay men". Its strategy indicates their perception of the nature and influence of churches and synagogues on American life and how they can be "turned around" to the point of view of the homosexual movement. In an interview which appeared in the National Gay Task Force's newsletter the campaign's director, Dr. Charles Hitchcock, was quite open about the project:

"Identifying key institutions which are central to the general public's understanding of social issues, educating staff in those organizations, and soliciting positive policies and support for gay rights from these groups is the heart of our agenda," stated Dr. Hitchcock. "We know from our breakthroughs in changing policies with both the American Psychiatric Association and the American Psychological Association that such programs can have a major impact on public attitudes, government policies, and our ability to achieve gay rights.

"Individual programs are being designed for each specific institution. Components include a history of each institution's attitudes or policies on gay rights, identification of institutional decision-makers and decision-making processes, and a curriculum for an educational (training) program with appropriate materials and resource people identified," he added. "A prime example would be that of a national television network where, because of the lack of any stated policy or educational materials concerned with gay issues, individuals are left to their own personal whim or prejudice in dealing with gay stories and news items. In targeting such an institution for our program, we would, through staff meetings, educational seminars and the development of relevant educational materials, hope to have a major positive impact on how that institution deals with gay concerns—both internally and in its entertainment programs and news coverage."

Churches, once they have been infiltrated by the homosexual movement, constitute one of its most important allies. Not only because of the ideological and human support they provide, but also on account of the availability of meeting rooms and other physical assets, the collaboration of churches can make the difference between the success and failure of a homosexual organizational activity. Thus readers are reminded that if they belong to a religious body—whether parish, congregation, or temple—their organization is of great interest to, indeed is a target of, the homosexual movement, which works relentlessly to take over its structures for its own purposes.

CHAPTER SIX

The Homosexual Movement and American Liberalism

There is little question that the homosexual movement is part and parcel of the American left.

This does not mean that liberals are homosexuals, that liberals necessarily accept the homosexual ideology, or that they actually sympathize with the movement. Nor does it mean that all liberal organizations do, in fact, support homosexuality. It does mean, however, that most homosexual organizations are an important component of the left-wing coalition.

As part of the research for this book, we conducted a survey of eighty randomly selected homosexual organizations. The results shows these organzations to be biased in favor of liberalism. The survey included questions on social, economic, and foreign policy issues, selected according to the public issues that were being widely discussed when the survey was undertaken. Table 4 shows the distribution of responses for each of the issues included in the survey.

In our survey, respondents were given three choices: agreement or disagreement with the policies or no opinion on the subject at all. The only issue on which homosexual organizations did *not* favor the liberal line was that of "block grants." This is easily explained by the fact that homosexual organizations have much more influence on local governments than they have on the federal govern-

TABLE 4

Opinions of Homosexual Organizations Concerning Public Policy Issues

Area	Agree			Disagree			No Opinion	
Social Issues	N	%		N	%		N	%
Family Planning Servies	73	91	*	2	2		5	6
Sex Education	78	98	*	0	0		2	2
Gun Control	66	82	*	12	15		2	2
ERA	76	95	*	2	2		2	2
Gay Rights	77	96	*	3	4		0	0
Family Protection Act	6	8		63	79	*	11	15
Abortion on Demand	76	95	*	1	1		3	4
Economic Issues								
Tax Cuts	42	53		30	36	*	8	10
Budget Cuts	6	8		65	81	*	9	11
Block Grants	28	35		24	30	*	28	35
Defense/Foreign Policy Issues								
Increased Military Spending	7	9		68	85	*	5	6
Dev. of Neutron Bomb	1	1		69	86	*	10	12
Military Aid to El Salvador	0	0		74	92	*	6	8

*Denotes liberal position on the issue.

ment. Since the effect of block grants is to shift the responsibility for allocating funds to the state and local bureaucracies, it is only natural that homosexual organizations would tend to support this policy. It is surprising, however, that in spite of the fact that block grants would mean such a budget increase, only 35% support them.

On a related issue, 53% of the organizations indicated support for tax cuts. This reflects in part the class com-

TABLE 5

Interpretation of Table 4

Descriptor	Range of Scores
Very Liberal	-7.16 to -10.00
Liberal	-4.29 to -7.15
Somewhat Liberal	-1.43 to -4.28
Neutral	$+1.42$ to -1.42
Somewhat Conservative	4.28 to 1.43
Conservative	7.15 to 4.29
Very Conservative	10.00 to 7.16

position of the homosexual community (that is, tax cuts would benefit homosexuals proportionately more than the rest of the population since they are wealthier). Moreover, both liberals *and* conservatives in the U.S. Congress were proposing tax cuts while the survey was under way. What is significant is that 36% were opposed to any tax cuts at all (whether proposed by liberal Democrats or President Reagan). Another significant figure is the 14% no-opinion response to the Family Protection Act issue. This probably reveals a lack of knowledge of the act. The 15% response on the conservative side of the gun control issue probably reflects the fear of crime among homosexuals resulting from their vulnerability, caused in turn by social conditions.

The scores in the three areas were converted to a linear scale, as was the total score. The total range on each area and the total were divided into seven categories with adequate descriptors. Table 5 shows the scores assigned to each descriptor.

Tables 6 through 9 show the number of homosexual organizations, their percentages, and cumulative percentages that belong to each of the political categories:

TABLE 6

Ideological Distribution of Homosexual Organizations: Overall Scores

Very Liberal	40	50%	50%
Liberal	32	40%	90%
Somewhat Liberal	5	6%	96%
Neutral	1	1%	97%
Somewhat Conservative	1	1%	98%
Conservative	1	1%	99%
Very Conservative	0	0%	99%
Total	80	99%	—

*Categories do not add up to 100% due to rounding.

TABLE 7

Ideological Distribution of Homosexual Organizations: Social Policy Issues

Very Liberal	73	91%	91%
Liberal	5	6%	97%
Somewhat Liberal	0	0%	97%
Neutral	0	0%	98%
Somewhat Conservative	1	1%	98%
Conservative	1	1%	99%
Very Conservative	0	0%	99%
Total	80	99%	—

*Categories do not add up to 100% due to rounding.

Table 6 reveals that 90% of the homosexual organizations are liberal or very liberal and that only 4% are either conservative or neutral. Fully 50% of the homosexual organizations are very liberal.

When social issues are considered by themselves, homosexual organizations are very liberal by an overwhelming majority. Moreover, they score consistently liberal on a variety of issues, indicating the pervasive acceptance of

TABLE 8

Ideological Distribution of Homosexual Organizations: Foreign Policy Issues

Very Liberal	60	75%	75%
Liberal	10	12%	87%
Somewhat Liberal	5	6%	93%
Neutral	2	3%	96%
Somewhat Conservative	3	4%	100%
Conservative	0	0%	100%
Very Conservative	0	0%	100%
Total	80	100%	—

*Categories do not add up to 100% due to rounding.

TABLE 9

Ideological Distribution of Homosexual Organizations: Economic Policy Issues

Very Liberal	11	14%	14%
Liberal	11	14%	28%
Somewhat Liberal	19	25%	53%
Neutral	15	18%	71%
Somewhat Conservative	16	20%	91%
Conservative	6	7%	98%
Very Conservative	2	2%	100%
Total	80	100%	—

liberal positions within the homosexual movement. From a political point of view, the implication of this phenomenon is that elected officials or candidates whose point of view is to the center or right of the center can expect little support (if not outright opposition) from homosexual groups.

In terms of foreign policy, homosexual organizations are also overwhelming liberal; 93% of them identify with leftist positions, only 4% are somewhat conservative, and none scored conservative or very conservative. This does not mean that all homosexuals are liberal on foreign policy, but that homosexual organizations agree with leftist positions. This can only be expected to translate into political action in support of organizations which have a specific interest in promoting leftist causes. These homosexual organizations can also be expected to become part of left-leaning networks.

The liberal make-up of the homosexual movement is obvious even in the area of economic policy. Although the survey was undertaken at a time when a wave of economic conservatism was sweeping America, over half the homosexual organizations proved to be liberal and less than one-third were in any way conservative. It is significant that 28% were distributed at the liberal-very liberal end of the scale while less than 10% were either conservative or very conservative.

It is not surprising that the homosexual movement is liberal on social policy issues. After all, the movement is centered on a membership trait whose acceptance implies a veritable revolution in the nation's laws and customs in family relationships, sex-related questions, feminism, and many other elements of the social policy area. The relations between the social policy and the economic and foreign policy components, however, have serious implications for the practictioner of politics.

Traditionally, profamily, prolife, and other social conservatives have taken issue with the homosexual movement, while foreign and economic policy conservatives have tended to skirt it on the basis that homosexuality per se has no bearing on foreign policy or economics. Indeed, there is no logical reason why a homosexual cannot agree with supply-side economics or a strong defense policy against the aggressive advance of communism in Central America. However, homosexuality (the sexual attraction for people of one's own sex) is not the same as the homosexual movement (a complex set of social institutions which accept and promote the homosexual ideology).

The defeat of the homosexual movement—as opposed to the mere "conversion" of homosexuals to celibacy or heterosexuality—is of great interest not only to social conservatives, but to *all* conservatives. Liberals have understood this well. Thus the homosexual movement enjoys their support and reciprocates their assistance whenever possible.

There are many, many ways in which American liberalism contributes to the ultimate goal of the homosexual movement—the acceptance of the "gay lifestyle" as part of American society and of homosexual acts as normal variants of human behavior. The following list summarizes these ways. Naturally some liberal politicians have contributed more to the homosexual movement than others. Many have avoided the issue altogether. However, there is myriad evidence that the several ways by which the liberal establishment contributes to the homosexual movement include:

—Promoting prohomosexual legislation
—Attacking profamily legislation
—Issuing orders or regulations which favor the homosexual movement
—Providing public funding for homosexual organizations
—Nominating avowed homosexuals for public positions
—Issuing declarations on the occasion of homosexual celebrations

—Participating in homosexual events: rallies, marches, etc.

—Meeting in their official capacities with leaders of the homosexual movement

—Hiring avowed homosexuals for their staffs

—Creating offices and positions to deal with homosexual questions in a way favorable to the homosexual movement.

In sum, the future of the homosexual movement rests, in part, on the future of American liberalism itself.

CHAPTER SEVEN

Goals of the Homosexual Movement

The ultimate goal of the homosexual movement can be summarized in a very simple phrase:

ACCEPTANCE OF HOMOSEXUAL ACTS AS A NORMAL VARIANT OF HUMAN BEHAVIOR AND OF HOMOSEXUALITY AS AN ALTERNATIVE LIFESTYLE

This goal obviously involves two distinct components. One refers to homosexual behavior and the other to the homosexual lifestyle. Although on the surface these are clear-cut notions, reality is not that simple. Homosexual behavior refers to the satisfaction of erotic desires by engaging in sexual activity with members of one's own sex. The homosexual lifestyle refers to the active and open practice of homosexuality, as well as to the attendant cultural patterns "typical" of the homosexual community. *America*, a Jesuit magazine, has articulated this objective in no uncertain terms:

> But the ultimate objective of at least a significant segment of the movement for homosexual rights is not simply to establish legal protection for homosexuals against any discrimination based on their private lives, but also to win eventual acceptance, on the part of both society and church, of homosexual behavior as a legitimate alternative that holds the full promise of human development and is in every way consistent with the Judeo-Christian ethical tradition.

Nearly all activities undertaken by the homosexual movement through its array of organizational components ultimately lead, directly or indirectly, to the accomplishment of this goal.

In some cases, this relationship is rather obvious. Organized groups of homosexuals within various professional associations lobby fiercely for "official declarations" by their parent organizations which resemble the dogmatic definitions of mainline churches. Organizations of homosexuals within churches seek justification in the Bible or the "evolving consensus of theologians" for the principle that homosexuality, if not individual homosexual acts, is perfectly within the order of nature. The concept of homosexual marriage, or "gay holy union"—widely accepted within the various homosexual religious communities—has been developed as a means of assimilating homosexual relationships into the accepted range of sexual relations among human beings.

Sex education centered on secular humanist principles rather than traditional morality has as one of its purposes to instill "toleration" and "understanding" in students for variant forms of "consensual" sexual behavior—that is, homosexuality. In addition, laws which imply the acceptance of homosexuals as a legitimate minority indirectly contribute to the acceptance of homosexuality. The imposition of "gayspeak" on the population frames the perception of the homosexual condition so as to make it impossible for the average user to conceive homosexuality as other than normal.

Activities within homosexual organizations—open sex in bathhouses, homosexual prostitution, open search for sex partners in bars, "cultural" events, and so forth—not only reinforce the homosexual condition in those affected by it, but accompany that reinforcement with principles and practices which, a least by implication, assert that homosexuality is normal. And, finally, the ideology of the homosexual movement is nothing but a set of principles which logically imply the normality of the homosexual condition.

The acceptance of homosexual behavior as normal implies not only the willingness to engage in social intercourse with individuals known or suspected to be homosexual, but the acknowledgment that when these individuals seek relief from their sexual urges they do so without violating their own nature. And the acceptance of homosexuality as an alternative lifestyle implies the extension of American cultural pluralism to areas that have been considered manifestations of depravity, emotional disorders, and/or sociopathic personalities.

Thus the primary goal of the homosexual movement is, in effect, a composite statement that implies a judgment on present mores and a substantial attack on the traditional values of American society. On the surface this would appear merely to broaden the scope of existing values (such as compassion, acceptance, understanding, pluralism, and so forth). In reality, it constitutes a radical challenge to established values and a demand that society redefine basic concepts which relate to sex as a core element in human personality.

Theoretically, it is possible for all homosexual organizations to work for the transformation of society by the accomplishment of a broad goal to which all can subscribe. In practice, however, this goal must be divided into smaller and more manageable tasks or subordinate goals. In each organization and in each geographic area, homosexual organizations endeavor to come closer to their ultimate purpose by attempting to accomplish a variety of goals depending on their specific needs or interest. Thus the North American Man/Boy Love Association works for the acceptance of transgenerational sex in law and as a permanent feature of our culture, while Dignity tries to have one Catholic diocese after another drop its opposition to "gay rights" legislation, or establish an official church organization to relate to homosexuals according to the tenets of their ideology.

In all cases, the final effect is the progressive transformation of society according to the homosexual conception, but each organization goes about this effort in its own peculiar way. Tradition-minded organizations opposed to society by the homosexual movement must be met according to the mode in which the challenge is posed. Otherwise, efforts to meet the challenge will be wasted and fail. It is only by understanding what the specific homosexual organization *really* intends, and why it goes about its efforts in such a peculiar way, that the issues presented can be framed in an intelligible and winnable manner. For example, once the principles of secular humanism are accepted within the framework of psychology, it is nearly useless to respond to the challenge posed by the homosexual movement in asserting that homosexuality is not a mental disorder. The total transformation of society by the acceptance of homosexuality as an alternative lifestyle and of homosexual acts as normal is evident in the "1972 Gay Rights Platform." Adopted by a National Coalition of Gay Organizations in February of that year, it constitutes one of the most detailed outlines of the homosexualized society produced thus far by the movement. Many of the elements of this list, considered in isolation, fall under specific categories within the various kinds of goals of the homosexual movement. But taken as a whole these demands provide the reader with a vision of what the ideal society sought by the homosexual movement would be:

1972 GAY RIGHTS PLATFORM

DEMANDS:
Federal:

1. Amend all federal Civil Rights Acts, other legislation and government controls to prohibit discrimination in employment, housing, public accomodations and public services.

2. Issuance by the President of an executive order prohibiting the military from excluding for reasons of their sexual orientation, persons who of their own volition desire entrance into the Armed Services, and from issuing less-than-fully-honorable discharges for homosexuality; and the upgrading to fully honorable all such discharges previously issued, with retroactive benefits.

3. Issuance by the President of an executive order prohibiting discrimination in the federal civil service because of sexual orientation, in hiring and promoting; and prohibiting discriminations against homosexuals in security clearances.

4. Elimination of tax inequities victimizing single persons and same-sex couples.

5. Elimination of bars to the entry, immigration and naturalization of homosexual aliens.

6. Federal encouragement and support for sex education courses, prepared and taught by Gay women and men, presenting homosexuality as a valid, healthy preference and lifestyle as a viable alternative to heterosexuality.

7. Appropriate executive orders, regulations and legis-

lation banning the compiling, maintenance and dissemination of information on an individual's sexual preferences, behavior, and social and political activities for dossiers and data banks.

8. Federal funding of aid programs of Gay men's and women's organizations designed to alleviate the problems encountered by Gay women and men which are engendered by an oppressive sexist society.

9. Immediate release of all Gay women and men now incarcerated in detention centers, prisons and mental institutions because of sexual offense charges relating to victimless crimes or sexual orientation; and that adequate compensation be made for the physical and mental duress encountered; and that all existing records relating to the incarceration be immediately expunged.

State:
1. All federal legislation and programs enumerated in Demands 1, 6, 7, 8, and 9 above should be implemented at the State level where applicable.

2. Repeal of all state laws prohibiting private sexual acts involving consenting persons; equalization for homosexuals and heterosexuals for the enforcement of all laws.

3. Repeal all state laws prohibiting solicitation for private voluntary sexual liaisons; and laws prohibiting prostitution, both male and female.

4. Enactment of legislation prohibiting insurance companies and any other state-regulated enterprises from discriminating because of sexual orientation, in insurance and in bonding or any other prerequisite to employment or control of one's personal demesne.

5. Enactment of legislation so that child custody, adoption, visitation rights, foster parenting, and the like shall not be denied because of sexual orientation or marital status.

6. Repeal of all laws prohibiting transvestism and cross dressing.

7. Repeal of all laws governing the age of sexual consent.

8. Repeal of all legislative provisions that restrict the sex or number of persons entering into a marriage unit; and the extension of legal benefits to all persons who cohabit regardless of sex or numbers.

While the ultimate stage of the homosexual society is not yet achieved, homosexual organizations continue pressing for other "subordinate" goals that will hasten the accomplishment of the ultimate goal. It is in this spirit that the homosexual struggle continues. These individual subordinate goals of the homosexual movement cover three general areas: ideological, political, and social. The following examples are offered to illustrated how the implementation of these goals contributes to the total breakdown of traditional mores and values:

IDEOLOGICAL GOALS

The fundamental ideological goal of the homosexual movement can be summarized in this simple phrase:

PROGRESSIVE ACCEPTANCE OF THE VARIOUS ELEMENTS OF THE HOMOSEXUAL IDEOLOGY

The total acceptance of the homosexual ideology in terms of social behavior would signify the complete identification of our culture with the homosexual subculture. Thus we must keep in mind the various activities or factors which contribute to the acceptance of the homosexual ideology. In some instances they act directly in making this acceptance possible; more often than not the effect is indirect, at times quite subtle. Included are:

—Continuing exposure to homosexual themes in the media, theater, and other modes of communication.

—Reorganization of the legal system to suit the requirements of the homosexual movement.

—Systematic affirmation of various propositions included in the homosexual ideology either directly or by implication.

—Use of inclusive language and/or practices which contribute to creating confusion in the roles of men and women within the family, church, economic units, governmental organizations, and so forth.

—Progressive weakening of family bonds by the institution of "open marriage," the increase and facilitation of divorce, the implementation of "children's rights," and so forth. (The concept of alternative family appears to be vital to the homosexual movement.)

—Continuing expansion of sexual subjectivism and moral relativism as acceptable tools for decision making, both within and without the sexual sphere.

—Acceptance and expansion of pornography as a "valid" expression of human feelings and/or a proper vehicle to satisfy a legitimate human need.

—Consistent utilization of expressions that imply the objectivity of the homosexual ideology (such as calling homosexuals "gay," homosexuals as a group a "minority," or homosexuality an "alternative lifestyle" rather than a disease or perversion).

POLITICAL GOALS

Certain subordinate goals of the homosexual movement can be logically classified as political in nature. This should not be surprising since the homosexual movement is fundamentally a political phenomenon. In general, the political goals of the homosexual movement pertain to the exercise of formal authority by the various jurisdictions of our political system.

Within the homosexual movement, no issue seems to have more importance than the passage of prohomosexual legislation. The universal features of these laws are: first, the acceptance of the principle that homosexuals constitute a legitimate minority; second, the concept that homosexuals have been unjustly discriminated against in the past and are thus entitled to special treatment under the law. In certain cases, this treatment extends to affirmative action programs in which homosexuals are actually preferred in the provision of services. Of course, this concept carries some danger for the homosexuals themselves, since it forces them to disclose the nature of their sexual preferences.

The National Gay Task Force monitors the programs of the homosexual movement and has produced—partly with the help of federal CETA Title VI funds—a classification of the various areas typically covered by prohomosexual laws. The following listing will acquaint the reader with these areas as described by the NGTF:

Employment means the provision or an offer to provide employment to an individual which includes opportunity for advancement based upon merit and/or other established criteria and including all benefits of employment.

Public Employment includes the above mentioned provisions for employment and in some specific cases requires that the City Manager (or other municipal) official include in all contracts, agreements and memoranda of understanding, the condition that contractors, in the performance of the contract, shall not discriminate on the basis of sexual orientation against any employee of, or applicant for employment with the contractor. Those contracts would extend and be applicable to all subcontracts.

Public Accommodations includes all services or facilities which are generally open to or offered to the public or which generally solicit public patronage or usage, whether operated for profit or not, e.g., theaters, hotels, retail stores, banks, hospitals, public conveyances, etc.

Housing describes any building or structure which is used or occupied or is intended, arranged, or designed to be used as a home, residence, or sleeping place of one or more individuals, groups or families, whether or not living independently of each other.

Education includes all public and private schools and training centers.

Real Estate Practices refers to exhibiting, listing, advertising, negotiating, agreeing to transfer, whether by sale, lease, sublease, rent assignment, or other agreement, any interest in real property or improvements upon that property.

Credit is defined as that credit which a person possesses as an individual and which is founded on the opinions held of their character or business standing. In many instances banking and insurance practices are also covered under the heading of "credit."

Union Practices refers to any person, employee representation committee or plan in which employees participate, or any agent or employee, which exists wholly or in part for the purpose of dealing with employers concerning grievances, labor disputes, wages, rates of pay, hours or other conditions of employment.

Affirmative Action Programs describes a bona fide plan designed to overcome the effects of past discrimination and to take action not otherwise prohibited by any other ordinance or state or federal law to carry out such an affirmative action plan.

One key area of legislative concern for the homosexual movement is the elimination of all legal restrictions on consensual sexual practices. Whether this elimination of legal restrictions is to apply to adults only or is also to be extended to minors depends on specific groups. Children's liberation organizations and "man/boy love" associations promote measures which eliminate transgenerational restrictions. In 1981 the Washington City Council was set to enact a measure which partially accomplished this goal (a committee of the council had actually approved such a bill!) when public pressure forced a change and a much "softer" bill was passed—only to be vetoed by the U.S. House of Representatives. For proponents of transgenerational sex, this is only a step toward a more comprehensive change in legislation.

The extent to which the goal of prohomosexual legislation in the United States has been successfully accomplished is considerable. The chart on the next page displays just a few of the jurisdictions in which a variety of prohomosexual measures have been enacted. It must be noted that many of these jurisdictions are "college towns" in which well-organized homosexual student groups have managed to impose prohomosexual legislation on the permanent residents. In many of the larger jurisdictions, prohomosexual measures are the result of "executive orders" in which local legislative bodies have not had the opportunity of voting the measures up or down. In several cases, homosexual behavior has been legalized by liberal courts which have declared laws banning sex between persons of the same sex illegal for a variety of reasons.

Prohomosexual Legislation in the United States (June 1981)

Municipality	Year(s) Enacted	Public Employment	Public Accommodations	Employment	Housing	Education	Real Estate Practices	Credit	Union Practices	Affirmative Action Program	Homosexual Acts
Alfred, N.Y.	5/74	X	X	X	X	X	X	X	X		
Amherst, Mass.	5/76	X	X	X	X	X	X	X	X		
Ann Arbor, Mich.	7/72	X	X	X	X			X	X		
Aspen, Colo.	11/77	X		X	X		X	X	X		
Atlanta, Ga.	7/71	X									
Austin, Tex.	7/75	X									
Berkeley, Calif.	10/78	X									
Bloomington, Ind.	12/75	X	X	X		X	X				
Boston, Mass.	4/76	X								X	
Champaign, Ill.	7/77	X	X	X	X			X	X		
Chapel Hill, N.C.	9/7	X									
Columbus, Oh.	1/79		X		X			X			
Cupertino, Calif.	2/75	X								X	
Detroit, Mich.	1/79	X	X	X	X	X	X	X			
East Lansing, Mich.	5/73	X	X	X	X						
Evanston, Ill.	8/80	X			X						
Hartford, Conn.	4/79	X		X							
Honolulu, Hawaii	3/81	X									
Iowa City, Iowa	5/77	X	X	X				X			
Ithaca, N.Y.	9/74	X								X	
Los Angeles, Calif.	5/77	X	X	X	X	X	X				
Madison, Wisc.	3/75	X	X	X	X		X				
Marshall, Minn.	4/75	X	X	X	X			X			
Milwaukee, Wisc.	7/80	X									
Minneapolis, Minn.	4/74	X	X	X	X	X	X	X	X		
Mountainview, Calif.	3/75	X								X	
New York, N.Y.	1/78	X									
Palo Alto, Calif.	8/74	X				X					
Philadelphia, Pa.	10/80	X									
Portland, Oreg.	12/74	X									
Pullman, Wash.	4/76	X			X					X	
San Francisco, Calif.	7/78	X	X	X	X						
Santa Barbara, Calif.	8/75	X				X					

SOURCE: "Gay Rights Protections in the U.S. and Canada," June 1981.

SOCIAL GOALS

There are a number of social goals espoused by the homosexual movement. These goals are designed to effect a transformation of social institutions and practices in harmony with the tenets of the homosexual ideology and the needs of the homosexual movement. The various social goals of the homosexual movement that we list here are merely by way of example, and are limited only by reasons of space. We hope and believe that these examples will be sufficient to illustrate the kind of society the homosexual movement intends to create in America.

In November 1979, the National Gay Task Force conducted a survey of its members, the results of which reveal the priorities of the very active and socially conscious membership of the NGTF. They include consensus on:

—The right of avowed homosexuals to be public school teachers

—Passage of the Equal Rights Amendment

—Adoption of children by homosexuals

—Passage of prohomosexual legislation

—Utilization of media to promote a positive image of homosexuals

—Elimination of "anti-gay" policies in federal agencies

—Utilization of the court system to advance the goals of the homosexual movement.

Homosexual organizations with a narrower focus, such as the North American Man/Boy Love Association, have their own blueprints and specific sets of activities for reshaping the United States to suit the sexual needs of its members. The following outline was published by the *NAMBLA Journal* as the social action agenda of the "Task

Force on Child-Adult Relations" (TFCAR). The general objectives of TFCAR are "to improve the social status and public image of pedophiles, to eliminate the legal sanctions against pedophile behavior, and to increase public awareness of children's emotional and sexual needs." The activities proposed for the TFCAR are all designed to bring these goals to fruition:

1. Seeking to improve the public image of pedophiles through:

A. Oversight of sex-education and psychology curricula in public schools, colleges, and universities, seeking to eliminate old stereotypes and falsehoods regarding pedophilia and children's sexuality.

B. Consultation with authorities on mental health and human sexual behavior to encourage a humane attitude toward pedophilia.

C. Legislative lobbying to reduce legal sanctions against pedophile behavior in particular and all consensual sexual behavior in general, and to increase children's rights to self-determination.

D. Liaison with feminist and other groups to establish the principle that the goals of all liberation groups are essentially the same: the elimination of sexist, authoritarian regimentation of human lives; and that the liberation of children is the *sine qua non* of all human liberation.

2. Publication and dissemination of literature supporting the goals of pedophile liberation.

3. Publication and dissemination of literature to increase public awareness of children's sexual and emotional needs, especially in the light of research on cognitive development.

This outline was proposed by a man imprisoned for child-molestation, who apologizes in this way for his inability to implement these plans: "I regret that I cannot do so at the present time because I am in prison for 'crimes' of pedophilia."

CONCLUSION

In sifting through the homosexual movement's various goals, it is clear that the movement's top priority is to force a "redefinition" of the American family away from the traditional husband-wife-children model to a more "functional" definition based on the notion of economic unit or any other basis that does not require heterosexuality as its foundation. Indeed, the notion that a family must involve persons of both sexes is profoundly inimical to the homosexual movement. After all, by their own definition heterosexual relations are beyond their reach; thus the traditional family as a normal institution for human relations is, to them, utterly unacceptable. This is why apologists for the homosexual movement—even those who otherwise profess allegiance to traditional beliefs—commonly join in the movement's attacks on the family as an institution.

The "new" family sought by the homosexual movement is certainly not one based on the traditional structure proposed by the Bible and enshrined by centuries of universal practice. In this "progressive" scheme, the natural foundation for family relations would disappear. In its place the autonomous self-defining will would be enshrined as sole subjective master.

Thus the ultimate goal of the homosexual movement is the transformation of key social structures and our entire culture according to the pattern dictated by the homosex-

ual ideology, to satisfy the individual needs of the homosexuals themselves—chiefly their sexual needs, but also the corporate needs of their organizations. Although not publicized widely, and normally unacknowleged, the foundation for a political and juridical system in which homosexuality is accepted as an alternative and legitimate lifestyle, and in which homosexual acts are not merely tolerated but positively accepted, requires the structural transformation of our society. It is a transformation the overwhelming majority of American would find repugnant.

Whether or not this transformation effort succeeds will depend not only on the skill and determination of the homosexual movement's leaders—but on the skill and determination of the majority of Americans to preserve traditional values as the foundation of society.

Additional information on the homosexual movement, with full documentation, is to be found in *The Homosexual Network*, by Enrique T. Rueda, published by Devin Adair, 680 pages. Available at $15.95 from Free Congress Foundation, 721 2nd Street, N.E., Washington, D.C. 20002, (202) 546–3004 or the Devin-Adair Company, 143 Sound Beach Avenue, P. O. Box A, Old Greenwich, Connecticut 06870, ~~(203) 637–4531~~.